9|10

# Joseph Christiano's

# BLOODTYPE

# Diet

## type

**A**

# Joseph Christiano's

# BLOODTYPE
# Diet
## type A

JOSEPH CHRISTIANO, ND, CNC

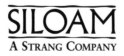

SILOAM
A STRANG COMPANY

Most STRANG COMMUNICATIONS BOOK GROUP products are available at special quantity discounts for bulk purchase for sales promotions, premiums, fund-raising, and educational needs. For details, write Strang Communications Book Group, 600 Rinehart Road, Lake Mary, Florida 32746, or telephone (407) 333-0600.

JOSEPH CHRISTIANO'S BLOODTYPE DIET, TYPE A
  by Joseph Christiano, ND, CNC
Published by Siloam
A Strang Company
600 Rinehart Road
Lake Mary, Florida 32746
www.strangbookgroup.com

Scripture quotations marked NKJV are from the New King James Version of the Bible. Copyright © 1979, 1980, 1982 by Thomas Nelson, Inc., publishers. Used by permission.

Cover design by Nathan Morgan
Design Director: Bill Johnson

Library of Congress Cataloging-in-Publication Data
Christiano, Joseph.
  Joseph Christiano's bloodtype diet, type A / by Joseph Christiano.
      p. cm.
  Includes bibliographical references.
  ISBN 978-1-61638-000-7
  1. Nutrition. 2. Blood groups. I. Title. II. Title: Bloodtype diet, type A.
  RA784.C513 2010
  612.1'1825--dc22
                                                    2010021065

*I would like to dedicate this book to my Creator and God, Yahweh. In His creative schemes for man's existence and mechanisms for survival, it never fails me how marvelously and wonderfully we are made in His likeness. With the capacities to love, hate, cry, laugh, worship, work, play, or a desire to excel into the unlimited heights that avail themselves to me in life's journey, all it takes is one minute of meditation on Him to be reminded of my total dependency on Him for all the provisions for my journey.*

# Acknowledgments

I WOULD LIKE TO thank Debbie Marrie for her willingness to work with me plus her constant flow of e-mails that served a great purpose in keeping me in line with all deadlines. For Barbara Dycus, whose lasting friendship makes every "work" a joy. And Tessie DeVore and the entire marketing team and editorial team members who, with their input and expertise, make this "work" another must-read.

I am grateful to Maria Gamb for her involvement in the dietary portion. Her expertise in matching and mixing the food groups, menus, and recipes for each blood type is greatly appreciated.

And without going unnoticed is my not-so-silent life partner, Lori. Her continual belief in me and what she sees in me has always given me that sense of worth. And always with a gentle push of confidence and pride she keeps me on my toes to write one more book. Thanks, babe. I love you!

# Contents

Introduction . . . . . . . . . . . . . . . . . . . . . . . . . . . . . . . 1

SECTION I: UNDERSTANDING BLOOD TYPES

1  Blood Types: Your Foundation for Health . . . . . . . . . 9
2  Blood Type and Nutrition . . . . . . . . . . . . . . . . . . . 19
3  Blood Type and Weight Loss . . . . . . . . . . . . . . . . . 33
4  Type A: Everything You Need to Know. . . . . . . . . . 45

SECTION II: THE BLOOD TYPE EATING PLAN

5  How to Become an Instinctive Eater . . . . . . . . . . . . 53
6  Getting Started: The Four-Week Test. . . . . . . . . . . 65
7  Individualized Eating Plan for Type A . . . . . . . . . . 75
8  Pick-a-Meal Recipes for Type A . . . . . . . . . . . . . . . 97
9  Nutritional Supplements for Type A . . . . . . . . . . . 135
10  Tips for Making It All Work . . . . . . . . . . . . . . . . . 153

    Appendix A: Nutrition Support Ideas . . . . . . . . . . 161
    Appendix B: Meal-Planner Chart. . . . . . . . . . . . . 166
    Appendix C: Thermoblast Weight-Loss
    Meal Replacements. . . . . . . . . . . . . . . . . . . . . . . . 167
    Appendix D: Thermoblast Twelve-Week
    Weight Loss Program . . . . . . . . . . . . . . . . . . . . . . 169
    Appendix E: Health and Fitness
    Coaching and Services . . . . . . . . . . . . . . . . . . . . . 171
    Appendix F: Services and Benefits . . . . . . . . . . . . 173
    Notes . . . . . . . . . . . . . . . . . . . . . . . . . . . . . . . . . . 175

# Introduction

SINCE WRITING THE book *Bloodtypes, Bodytypes, and You*, I cannot count the many people who have told me they improved their lives by applying the information it contains and changing their lifestyles. Many have said they experienced significant drops in their cholesterol and blood pressure readings. Others are saving hundreds of dollars on monthly medication costs because they have been able to reduce and/or completely eliminate taking medications. And they are delighted with the improvement in the way they are feeling. People have shared how they no longer are experiencing digestive disorders and associated discomfort—all because they started eating for their blood type and made other healthy lifestyle changes.

In addition to making food selections that are compatible to your blood type for improved illness profiles, increased energy levels, and help in reaching your ideal weight for life, I have included some additional information in this book that further unlocks the secrets to owning natural health and keeping weight off for life.

Did you know that one in three American adults (over 58 million) ages twenty to seventy-four is overweight?[1] Being overweight and physically inactive accounts for more than 300,000 premature deaths each year in the United States, second only to tobacco-related deaths.[2]

Due to the many requests of my readers, along with my

personal interest in helping people lose weight and *keep it off,* I have included a chapter dedicated to losing weight, helping you to reach your ideal weight for life. My weight-loss program focuses on enlisting help from your metabolism, learning how to rev it up so your body can do all the work by becoming the natural calorie burner it was designed to be.

This weight-loss protocol includes everyday meal plans that are compatible for blood type A. It also includes temporary meal-replacement snacks that are natural fat burners to jump-start the weight-loss process and eventually lead you into eating food (blood-type compatible) to reach your ideal weight for life.

My personal and professional experience for more than forty years in the field of health and fitness has shown me the most common denominator shared by dieters who lose weight: 95 percent of them gain all the weight back and more! Because so much emphasis is placed on dieting the weight off instead of eating foods that work in harmony with one's unique body chemistry, the failure rate remains extraordinarily high.

Life is precious and was given as a gift to you—free of charge. What you do with this extraordinary gift has direct conse-quences on every aspect of your life. As our world continually advances in technology, information, and new discoveries, can you honestly say that you are improving and moving in step with the areas of your life that mean the most? Consider the areas over which you have control, like personal relationships, happiness and contentment, and vibrant health and youthful, functional age. Why not choose to keep in step with accurate eating so that you can maintain your energy, your health, and your ideal weight for life? Have you made these goals a part of your lifestyle?

As you read this book, ask yourself this question: *Does my lifestyle contribute to or take away from these vital areas of my life?* Remember, you are responsible for making the right choices!

## Dr. Joe—Your Coach

As you and I establish a one-on-one relationship throughout this book, I want you to relate to me as Dr. Joe, your personal health and fitness life coach. My role will be to show you how to maximize the benefits of specific food selections that are most compatible for your blood type.

So, as Dr. Joe, your personal health and fitness life coach, it is my job to get you to where you want to go just as quickly as possible. Normally, if you hired me, I would ask you a series of background questions related to your medical history, diet experiences, and fitness goals. I would want to know as much about you as possible so I could prescribe the most beneficial strategies to reach your goals. Then I would provide you with a dietary program designed specifically to meet your individual nutritional needs.

This book will help you to develop such a dietary program. By teaching you the right foods for your blood type, I will help you to reach and maintain your healthy body weight, improve bodily functions, heal your body systems, reduce the likelihood of disease, control blood sugar, and improve metabolic function. I will have you fill out a dietary analysis of the foods and fluids you consume and the dietary supplements that can help you experience optimal health.

This book, which has been geared specifically for those with blood type A, is the closest thing to having your own nutrition coach—and a whole lot less expensive. The book is designed to implement my expertise through eating programs and information for your specific blood-type needs.

Naturally, the success of our modified version of one-on-one training will depend on how you apply the contents of this book. The synergy of our relationship through this book will take you to a new level of understanding of the importance of proper diet to benefit you most. Your adherence to your strategies will speed up the time for accomplishing your short- and long-range goals. It will also give you a greater sense of value in making this approach to a healthier you and a lifetime of vibrant living.

## From Me to You

Have you ever noticed the increased performance of your car engine when you fill the gas tank with high-octane fuel instead of low-octane fuel? The answer is obvious. The engine runs poorly on low-octane fuel. It interferes with the engine's performance. When you use high-octane fuel, your engine will perform more efficiently and smoothly. The drive will be faster because the higher octane is what your engine requires.

The same principle is true about the fuel you use in your body's "engine." By applying the higher-octane dietary strategies that are compatible to your genetics, you will enjoy the positive results sooner.

Having been an avid proponent of getting regular exercise, eating healthily, and taking nutritional supplements for most of my life, what I share in this book will come from my own personal and professional experiences over forty years. My own journey for finding better ways of achieving a more healthy, balanced life has caused my innate curiosity and desire to search beyond the mundane for more accurate and direct paths to optimum health.

I travel all over the country speaking and sharing the benefits that come from taking care of the body. I also work at staying in shape; I didn't just wake up one morning to discover I was in good shape—so we share the same journey. My personal level of fitness is a result of years of regular exercise, eating for my blood type, taking nutritional supplements, getting proper rest, and maintaining a positive mental attitude, a zeal for life, and faith in Yahweh (God)—my lifestyle.

But when I look at my daughters and the twelve grandchildren they have given me, I think about the positive role I can play in their lives. I value my relationship with my wife, and I know the importance a healthy body and mind have in our relationship. I look at other family members and wonder what it would be like if I were too sick to enjoy the time I spend with them.

No, maintaining my health is not a mechanical function to me. My good health didn't just happen. I have to work hard to get it—and to keep it. So will you. You will need to look beyond the sweat and discipline and focus on the really important things in your life, weighing them against an unhealthy and sickly lifestyle. I wrote a mantra that I follow, and I want you to consider it when it comes to getting the job done: "Focus on the purpose, not the task." I hope you will see the value in the principles in this book.

These new findings are important to adapt to our lifestyles so that faster results and responses for positive bodily performance can be achieved. Throughout the years, I have learned to make it a point to be more open-minded and willing to accept new truths and information that become available to me. This open-mindedness can be applied to diet, exercise, personal relationships, and my spiritual life—or to any area of my life. New research and studies are constantly being made available, so it would be foolish not to take the opportunity to become more informed. Such information can enhance your life and provide the impetus for continual progress.

So, if you haven't done anything to improve your health, or maybe you began and got lazy but realize it is time to take control again, I strongly encourage you to put into practice the strategies, guidelines, and new information you read in this book. Just reading about them cannot bring you a healthier lifestyle. Change will require *the will to change.*

If you are serious about discovering a healthy way of eating and if you want to live an energetic and youthful life that is high on performance and low on maintenance, then now is the time to make your decision. The journey will never end if you will remember that you are an inspiration in constant transition. Let's take the journey together—one-on-one!

# SECTION I

# UNDERSTANDING
# BLOOD TYPES

# Chapter 1

## BLOOD TYPES: YOUR FOUNDATION FOR HEALTH

D NA. Genome. Cellular profiling. Stem cells. Cloning. Blood types. What is it all about? Is the existence and physiological makeup of humankind just a mixture of theories, personal points of view, and yet-to-be proven truths? Are we dabbling into mysterious areas that should be left alone, or are we finally beginning to learn more about ourselves?

In man's conquest to survive, questions arise every day: What role do genes play in determining health, disease, longevity, bodily function, and performance? What is the origin of man—where did he come from? Do we all come from one main gene pool, or are we descendants of individual generational ancestry? Did we evolve from nothing to crawling on all fours to an eventual upright position, or did Yahweh (God's proper and personal name) create us? Is man degenerating because of cellular mutation, becoming less than what he started out as, or is he a result of an evolutionary process, making him far superior to what he was at the beginning of time? Why do some people enter life with blue eyes and blond hair and others with brown eyes and brown hair? Are certain body genetics designed for physical and athletic superiority while other body genetics determine the run-of-the-mill hopefuls? Do the ABO blood types react differently to the same foods? Is there a link between red blood cells and your health?

Although phenomenal advancements have been made through modern-day discoveries in technology, science, and medicine, it will still take eternity to unravel the amazing intricacies of man. The world's best scientific minds have made amazing discoveries, but in the light of all that we still do not know about ourselves, technology seems to move at a snail's pace.

Whether you believe that Yahweh created every human being or that our existence is a result of some theoretical development of nothingness into something, the answers to our questions lie far beneath the surface—with our genetic foundation.

Our genetic makeup is the foundation of all that is life. Nothing relating to our ability to survive our environment; to fight off illness, infection, or stress; to supply our bodies with nutrition; or to make physiological adaptation is a matter of happenstance. It is no coincidence that our bodies are programmed with the innate ability to defend us from uninvited invaders such as parasites, viruses, and bacteria by creating an army of antibodies.

Our genetic foundation is a mixture of trillions of cells with codes that identify, program, and link everything in our existence—the color of our hair, our bodies' susceptibility to disease, and foods that are compatible to our potential life span and capability to survive.

Some people would rather merely swim in shallow water than go below the surface to discover answers to the questions and issues of life. But there is a bottomless sea to dive into for the inquisitive and health-conscious individual who seeks knowledge of the role genetics play in our lives.

For example, did you know that...

- Gene therapy is now being researched intensively in most developed countries—for a host of very good reasons. Instead of treating deficiencies by injecting drugs, doctors will be able to prescribe genetic treatments that will induce the body's own protein-making machinery to produce the proteins needed to combat illness.[1]

- Researchers succeeded in making artificial copies of human genes that could be manipulated to produce large amounts of specific proteins. Such genes can be introduced into the human body where, in many cases, they substitute for a defective gene.[2]

- In a study that could lead to new treatments for diabetes and provide guidance on the use of genes in treating disease, scientists show that a common genetic variation increased the risk of contracting type 2 diabetes.[3]

- Australian scientists have identified a new gene responsible for controlling appetite in humans—a discovery experts say could lead to the first gene-based drug to treat obesity and diabetes.[4]

- In the not-too-distant future, scientists may be able to grow replacement organs and new blood vessels to replace clogged ones, eradicate diseases as diverse as Alzheimer's and cystic fibrosis, and tell which medication to prescribe.[5]

Gaining more knowledge and understanding about the complexities of our genetics humbles me—and convinces me of the existence of One much greater than man, with infinite creative wisdom that stretches far beyond the finite knowledge of man. The fact that man has the ability to make scientific advancements and acquire information about the genome of man serves only to prove how much greater his Creator must be.

## The Discovery of Blood Groups

I also find it amazing that what the majority of us now know about our genetic makeup has only been discovered in recent decades. Experiments with blood transfusions began centuries ago, but without an understanding that there are different blood groups (also called blood types) many people died. At that time, no one knew that the blood clumping (*agglutination*), which caused toxic reactions and even death after some transfusions, was the result of mixing blood from two people with different blood types.

Then in 1901, an Austrian named Karl Landsteiner discovered that blood clumping was an immune system reaction that occurs when the receiver of a blood transfusion has antibodies that war against the donor's blood cells. His discovery led to the classification of different blood groups, making it possible to conduct blood transfusions much more safely. Landsteiner was awarded the Nobel Prize in 1930 for making this remarkable, life-saving discovery.

So, what is it about the blood that makes one blood group different from another? The differences in our blood are based on the presence or absence of antigens and antibodies. Antigens are located on the surface of the red blood cells, and antibodies are in the blood plasma. People have different types and combinations of these molecules, which are inherited from their parents.

There are more than twenty blood group systems known today, but since the ABO system is the one most people are familiar with, I'll stick with the ABO blood group system for our discussion of blood types in this book. As you're probably aware, according to the ABO system, there are four different kinds of blood groups: A, B, AB, and O.

### Blood group A

Since you purchased this book, I assume you belong to blood group A. As a member of this blood group, you have A antigens on the surface of your red blood cells and B antibodies in your blood plasma.

### Blood group B

People in this blood group have B antigens on the surface of their red blood cells and A antibodies in their blood plasma.

### Blood group AB

People in this blood group have both A and B antigens on the surface of their red blood cells and no A or B antibodies at all in their blood plasma.

### Blood group O

People in this blood group have neither A nor B antigens on the surface of their red blood cells, but they have both A and B antibodies in their blood plasma.

## How Did Different Blood Types Occur?

People who believe in Creation often ask: How did such a variety of ethnic groups and diverse races arise from one human pair?

Research is revealing more and more about the origin of blood types. Much of this research points out the possibility of the emergence of all known blood types from our common ancestors, Adam and Eve. In his dissertation titled "Blood Types and Their Origin (Answering the Critics)," Jonathan Sarfati tells us:

> There is one gene in humans that controls the ABO blood type. There are three versions of the gene, or alleles: A, B, or O.... For a husband and wife to pass on all alleles to their children, they need to, between them, have the A, B, and O alleles.... If Adam and Eve were genetically AO and BO, for example, their children could have had AB, AO, BO, or OO genetic makeup, giving AB, A, B, or O blood types. Indeed, about 25 percent of their children would have been of each type.[6]

There is so much more to be discovered about man and our genetic makeup—birthed in us at the moment of conception. Although scientists are discovering new things about our genetic structure daily, there is much more that remains unknown. One scientist has observed:

> Data supporting the complexity and design of life at all levels, and especially that of man, loom larger than was previously supposed—as large in fact as the enormous "gaps" in the fossil record.... The further we look into the complexity to the real world of man and his living companions, the more baffling and unexplainable, at

least in standard evolutionary theory, the whole complex becomes.... To the skeptic, the proposition that the genetic programmes of higher organisms consisting of something close to a thousand million bits of information... containing in encoded form countless thousands of intricate algorithms controlling, specifying, and ordering the growth and development of billions and billions of cells into the form of a complex organism, were composed by a purely random process is simply an affront to reason.[7]

It has taken gifted scientists years upon years to discover the things they know about man today. But it will take hundreds of more years to understand how to apply the new information.

It is when we are willing to be taught and are open to more knowledge that we continue to grow. I am growing daily in my own knowledge, particularly in my knowledge about the link between blood types and nutrition. Since authoring the book *Bloodtypes, Bodytypes, and You*, I have discovered new studies about the origin of blood types. These findings lean more closely to my personal beliefs in creationism.

My purpose for mentioning this is twofold: First, I humbly admit that no one has all the answers. But as long as we are willing to be open to greater learning and understanding, progress can be continual. Second, since I happen to believe that Yahweh is the Creator of all creation, it stands to reason that I would embrace studies that line up with my beliefs. As we learn more about the complex design of man, it just makes good sense to me that Someone greater than you or I is in charge of this whole thing.

Regardless of where you stand concerning the origins of blood type, one thing we can agree on is that eating foods compatible to our blood type and avoiding foods that are not compatible is a more accurate and individualized approach to eating than anything man has experienced.

As a naturopathic doctor, and not a scientist, biochemist, or genealogist, I'll leave the research and discoveries to them and concentrate my efforts on helping you to be healthier. My interest is to help you reach a basic level of understanding about your body so you can take care of it in a way that will contribute to living a healthier and more balanced life.

During my summer vacations from school as a kid, I remember going with my father while he worked a few hours a week for my cousin, who owned an excavation and construction company. I watched the construction workers build the foundations for new buildings, or as they called it, "pour a cellar." It was quite a process. The first thing they did was excavate the land and prepare the ground. Then they measured out the area where the foundation would be laid. After determining the proper elevations and measurements, they began to set up the forms.

Until I saw the entire process completed for the first time, it was hard to understand why they were using all those heavy planks to make a huge square in the dirt. But I learned that those planks played a very important role in the next part of the procedure. When the huge cement trucks were ready to pour the concrete, they poured it into the wood forms, which shaped the foundation of the building.

I learned that each foundation differed in size, shape, and materials. Certain job sites required the forms to be dug deeper in the ground, while other forms were extended higher. The deeper or higher the forms were laid, the thicker the concrete base or foundation would be. The design and composition of each poured foundation determined the size and weight of the structure that it could support.

Each building structure, whether a residential home, a high-rise building, or a strip mall, required a unique foundation that functioned as its basis for structure, stability, and support. Similarly, our ability to survive, support, and improve our structure will be determined by the mixture of the material found in our foundation. Our foundation, of course, is our genetics.

Consider yourself as a general contractor who wants to redesign or custom-build a house. In this case, the foundation of the house you want to construct, or reconstruct, is your genetics. Instead of brick, mortar, and wood, you are using the materials that comprise your body.

The amount of time and effort you put into customizing and building your "house" (your body) will help it to last for many years. By understanding the purpose of a strong "foundation" (your genetics) and by using the proper "tools and materials" (the proper nutritional and exercise applications and methodologies), you can assure a healthy, happy future.

You have a specific biological makeup that was given to you at conception. It's the genetic substance that makes up your entire existence.

I have three daughters—Amy, the oldest, and twin daughters, Jenifer and Cara. Amy's genetic foundation has given her facial features that resemble mine, while genetically Jenifer and Cara have their mother's facial features.

But your genes are not limited to your facial characteristics. Your genes not only determine if you will look more like your mom or your dad and what color your hair and eyes will be, but also how susceptible you are to certain diseases and illnesses.

Your cellular profile and the way your body responds to certain foods, viruses, and bacteria are determined by your genes also.

One very important consideration can greatly help you maximize your genetic potential. This is providing your body with the best nutritional program for your specific genetics. Let's take a look at this consideration in the next chapter.

## RECAP

To understand the importance of your blood type, remember the following:

1. All of us are made up of trillions of cells. We function by our cells.

2. Our genetic foundation can help us determine today and tomorrow how to prepare ourselves for potential illnesses and diseases.

3. Understanding the role our genetics (blood type) play will help individualize the dietary remedies we need to improve survival.

4. Your body at the cellular level responds differently to the same foods than other blood types may.

# Chapter 2

# BLOOD TYPE AND NUTRITION

I N THIS CHAPTER I will discuss the benefits of eating for your blood type, the importance of whole, unprocessed foods, and how to make this ideal a reality in your life. You've probably heard the saying, "You are what you eat," but I believe it is also vitally important that "you eat what you are"! Each of us should eat a diet that is compatible with our blood type.

We can begin to get an understanding of this important concept by taking a look at the animal kingdom. It is instinct that drives animals to eat. Lions are meat eaters—they won't be happy if you try to feed them a diet rich in fruits and vegetables. Other animals are vegetarian by instinct, and they will not eat meat. This is no accident—instinct is a protective mechanism for all animals, including humans.

Each blood type has different characteristics that allow it to eat, digest, and assimilate food best for that group. As a blood type A individual, you represent 40 percent of the population and are not designed to digest, assimilate, and utilize some of our country's food staples as red meat and potatoes. Because of your genetics, a safeguard of avoiding certain foods will greatly protect you from potential cardiovascular diseases that are common for your blood type. Type Os are blessed with strong stomach acid and powerful enzymes that can metabolize almost anything—even some of the foods that are not recommended for their blood type. Types A, B, and AB must be more careful in their eating habits or suffer the consequences.

What are these consequences? What happens when you eat food not compatible with your blood type? *Agglutination* (the blood clumping I mentioned in chapter 1) happens. Agglutination can be explained in more detail as follows:

> Your body has antibodies that protect it from foreign invaders. Your immune system produces all kinds of antibodies to protect you and keep you safe from foreign substances. Each antibody is designed to attach itself to a foreign substance or antigen. When your body recognizes an intruder, it produces more antibodies to attack the invader. The antibody then attaches itself to the intruder, and a "gluing" effect (agglutination) takes place. In this way, the body can better dispose of these foreign invaders.[1]

When it comes to eating foods that are not compatible with your blood type, this "gluing" effect can take place in the digestive system, joints, liver, brain, or blood. Continual ingesting of foods not compatible to your blood type can cause havoc in your body systems. This agglutination of cells, or clumping, will eventually break down the function of that particular system and lead to health problems.

You will find as you read on in this book that I identify certain foods as "avoid" foods. One reason for this is because of the protein molecules, or *lectins*, that they contain. When these dietary lectins that are present in certain foods enter your body, problems prevail.

Conversely, with proper diet, including nourishment from the food and supplements specific to your needs, the chance of disease is greatly reduced. In fact, proper diet according to blood type, coupled with exercise, enables your immune system to be its strongest. A strong immune system can make the difference between a longer or shorter life span.

## THE BASICS OF GOOD NUTRITION

For the rest of this chapter I will discuss the basics of good nutrition, but added to these basics will be the customized advice for your individual blood type. The basic guidelines to remember are simple:

- All foods you choose should be compatible with your blood type.

- Eat more protein than carbohydrates to keep your body in an anabolic state and your glycemic index as low as possible.

- Complex carbohydrates should be preferred over simple carbohydrates.

- Decrease saturated fats. Use blood type–appropriate monounsaturated and polyunsaturated fats instead.

- Eat a minimum of one to three large servings of dark leafy vegetables (such as kale, chard, collard greens, mustard greens, dandelion greens, or arugula) each day. The variety will depend upon your blood type requirements.

- Eat unprocessed foods whenever possible. Choose fresh foods.

- Eat organic foods whenever possible.

- Drink plenty of water (alkaline).

## Protein, the Anabolic State, and the Glycemic Index

Since the body cannot repair itself without protein, protein is the key element in the equation for good health. Blood type A individuals likewise require a generous amount of daily protein for many reasons. The source of your protein differs from the likes of your blood type O friends, as you are not predisposed to breakdown the heavy protein food sources that they can. Ideally, you want to get your proteins from vegetables and certain meats such as turkey, chicken, fish, and so on.

Every time you eat protein, the body produces glucagon and enters an anabolic state. This is the same state that happens when we abstain from excessive carbohydrates. Glucagon shifts the body into a burning mode. Proteins are converted to ketones, which are utilized for energy. Fat is released from the cells to be used as energy. The kidneys release excess water. Weight loss is the result.

Conversely, a catabolic state is when carbohydrates are converted to sugar in your body. The pancreas secretes insulin to keep the sugar levels in balance. The excess insulin places your body into a catabolic state. Catabolic state simply means that the insulin converts the protein into fats. These fats then are stored, resulting in excess weight. Another by-product of excess insulin production is the increase of cholesterol. The kidneys retain excess fluids, and glucose (sugar) is used as energy instead of fat. If our bodies are in a continual catabolic state, we subject ourselves to the risk of heart disease, high blood pressure, high cholesterol, and many other health problems.

Bear in mind that when we talk about protein, we are referring to lean, good-quality animal protein, fish, tofu, tempeh, and some legumes. Whenever possible it is advisable to consume organic or free-range animal products. These animal products are free from antibiotics, bovine growth hormones, steroids, and other sundry chemical residues. While these products may cost slightly more, it is important to remember that the quality of the food you put into your body is just as important as the specific types. It is not my intention to endorse high-fat protein sources, which will cause untold troubles for all readers.

Refer to the food list in chapter 7 for the specific dietary sources of protein I recommend for type A. To purchase protein powder compatible with type A, see Appendix A.

## Complex Carbs vs. Simple Carbs

There is a definite difference in which types of carbohydrates cause a catabolic state. Simple carbohydrates such as white bread, wheat bread, and rice cakes enter the bloodstream at a rapid rate. Foods such as these have a high glycemic index rating. Other complex carbohydrates such as cherries, apples, peanuts, soybeans, peaches, and rye bread enter the bloodstream much more slowly, thus resulting in a lower glycemic index rating. The slower the introduction into the bloodstream, the better. Please refer to the glycemic index chart on the next page to gain a better understanding of this principle. Understanding

## Glycemic Index of Common Foods

| | |
|---|---:|
| Cereals | 100+ |
| Puffed rice, rice cakes, puffed wheat | 133 |
| Maltose | 110 |
| Glucose | 100 |
| White bread, whole-wheat bread | 100 |
| Carrots | 92 |
| Oat bran, rolled oats | 88 |
| Honey | 87 |
| White rice, brown rice, corn, bananas | 82 |
| All Bran, kidney beans | 72 |
| Raisins, macaroni, beets | 64 |
| Pinto beans, sucrose | 59 |
| Peas, potato chips, yams | 51 |
| Sweet potatoes, sponge cake | 46 |
| Oranges, navy beans, grapes, 100% rye bread | 40 |
| Nonfat yogurt | 39 |
| Tomato soup | 38 |
| Apples, chickpeas, ice cream, yogurt, milk | 35 |
| Lentils, peaches | 29 |
| Cherries, grapefruit, plums | 25 |
| Soybeans | 15 |
| Peanuts | 12 |
| Juice ratings: | |
|     Peach, plum, cherry, grapefruit | Low |
|     Pear, orange, apple, grape | Moderate |
|     Banana | High |

the application of the glycemic index and which carbohydrates are best suited for you is very important. Whether your goal is to lose weight, help stabilize sugar, or combat hypoglycemia and diabetes, choose the lower GI numbers for best results. Examples of those lower-rated numbers are nonfat yogurt, peas, cherries, soybeans, and peanuts.

## The Fat Issue

Saturated fats are primarily derived from animal sources and rarely from plants. One characteristic of animal saturated fats is that when stored at room temperature, they solidify. Examples would be meat, butter, and cheeses. The common store-bought plant saturated fats you might recognize are coconut oil, peanut oil, cottonseed oil, and palm kernel oil. There is a close association of cholesterol-related health issues with these types of fats, including potential obstruction of arteries, which could cause heart failure. Studies suggest that excessive saturated fat consumption is also linked to some forms of cancer. Monounsaturated and polyunsaturated oils do not promote the accumulation of cholesterol in the arteries, as do the highly saturated fats. One of the best examples of these less destructive oils can be found in olive oil. Olive oil is the highest in monounsaturated fats available. In our "fat-crazed" society we tend to forget to differentiate saturated fats from monounsaturated and polyunsaturated fats. So enjoy that dressing you made with heart-friendly olive oil! Eating the right fats should be high on your list of healthy lifestyle choices.

Several oils are compatible for all blood types and thus can be shared equally. Your ideal or most beneficial fats would be linseed, flaxseed, and olive oils. Next would be canola and cod liver oils. You may want to include compatible nuts and seeds for their oil values as well as their values in protein.

## GREEN LEAFY VEGETABLES

Dark leafy green vegetables such as kale, chard, collard greens, mustard greens, dandelion greens, and arugula are especially important to mention. These vegetables have a host of benefits for everyone. They improve digestion of fats and proteins and improve circulation. Mustard greens in particular aid in dissolving stagnant or congealed blood. Dark leafy greens are considered the "blood cleaners" of the vegetable kingdom. They provide much-needed chlorophyll, which inhibits viruses and colds. Vitamin A, vitamin C, and calcium are also part of the benefits. Some are rich in fiber as well. Women who are concerned about getting enough calcium should try eating an extra serving of these healthy greens. Refer to the food list in chapter 7 for the specific dietary sources of protein I recommend for type A.

It's interesting that the color of vegetables says a lot about their characteristics, but there's a lot more to the story. If you want to drop a few pounds, vegetable oils help prevent water retention. So including them will assist in weight loss or in maintaining your ideal weight. Keeping your plate full of compatible vegetables is great weight management strategy. Blood type As always do well with vegetable proteins as they are easy to digest and utilize. Of course, the nutritional values from veggies, either steamed, raw, or slightly seared, assist in supplying your nutritional requirements and satisfying those hungry taste buds.

## Unprocessed, Fresh, and Organic Foods

Eating healthily can sometimes be daunting given the current advertising environment in this country. There are plenty of people touting that this product or that product is the best. But in the end, most fall short of being healthy or nutritious at all. We as Americans consume vast quantities of processed foods laden with sugar, fats, and highly processed wheat. Items touted as "fat free" should be a warning signal to each of us. In order for a product to be tasty yet fat free, the manufacturer will boost the sugar content. Sucrose, which is the standard white table sugar, contributes to diabetes, hypoglycemia, and many other ailments. However, the point here is that there is nothing in these foods you really need. Products that are "fortified" or "enriched" are merely attempts to put back into the food that which has been processed out. Type A individuals are genetically predisposed to having tissue sensitivities. Certain stressors can cause your sensitive tissues to become acidic. Keeping an eye on what type of activities you choose and the amount of stress you are under may help prevent a pH imbalance. Yoga, circuit training, and stretching are great activities. Emotional stressors also play havoc on your pH levels, so relaxation methods, prayers, walking, singing, deep breathing exercises, and just plain ol' "chillin'" really work well for you in combating pH imbalance.

In my humble opinion, it's best to wipe the slate completely clean when it comes to processed foods. All the vitamins, minerals, and nutrients you need can be found in simple, fresh produce. Again, the important factor is that you are making an investment in yourself. *You* are your most valuable asset. So the quality of what you put into your body is vitally important.

We covered organic and free-range animal products earlier. There are also organic vegetables, fruits, and virtually every other kind of produce you can imagine. For something to be organic, it has to be free of toxic chemical insecticides, fungicides, pesticides, and herbicides. There is a tremendous difference in taste between an organic carrot and one harvested by traditional methods. Just try it! But more important than the taste is the basic principle of not putting anything laden with chemicals into your body.

If organic products are not available in your area or are undesirable to you, the next best thing would be to buy from local farmers. Most cities host some phenomenal fresh markets. If you are unsure of where to find a fresh market, contact your local Department of Agriculture. Farmers boast both traditional and organic produce. By buying from the farmers direct, you are insuring that you are getting the freshest produce possible, thereby giving you the maximum amount of vitamins and minerals. Also, you are avoiding the extra chemicals and waxing that is used to preserve the produce in transit to large grocery stores.

If you prefer the convenience of ordering online, see Appendix A for a list of sites that can provide you with a variety of dried goods from grains, pastas, and legumes to condiments.

## Tracking What You Eat

Now that you are beginning to see the importance of eating foods that are beneficial to your blood type and avoiding foods that are toxic, I would like to recommend that you track what you eat for a few days. Most of us don't realize the amount of little tastes or little bites of food we consume throughout each day—especially of foods that we should avoid. As you track your eating, you will be amazed at how far off the mark you may have been—and yet you never saw it happening.

Use the dietary analysis chart on page 32 to track your eating. For three consecutive days, simply record everything you eat and drink. Record the time you eat each meal or snack. Record the number of cups of coffee and/or cans of soda. If you eat a cookie or have a bowl of ice cream, write down an accurate record of what you ate.

## THREE RULES OF HEALTHY EATING

1. Eat when you are hungry.

2. Eat until you are satisfied (not stuffed).

3. Hit the brakes if you are eating when you are not hungry. It's emotional, and you cannot resolve emotional issues through your plate of food.

Your dietary analysis will give you an accurate account of whether you are consuming foods that are compatible for your blood type. It will also help you to stay on track. If I were your personal trainer, I would be asking you dietary questions all the time. Tracking your diet will make a big difference in your success or failure—especially when you hit a plateau.

Food can work for you or against you, as we have seen. It can stimulate weight loss, or it can cause weight gain. If weight loss is your goal, take a look at the weight loss/gain lists for blood type A on page 97.

Whether weight loss is your focus or not, the dietary analysis chart on page 32 is best to use before you start out on your journey. That way you get a realistic look at your present eating habits. As you proceed through your exercise journey, repeat the dietary analysis as often as you feel the need to double-check yourself.

## Recap

The basic guidelines for my blood types' eating plans are simple:

1. All foods you choose should be at least 80 percent compatible with your blood type.

2. Eat more protein than carbohydrates to keep your body in an anabolic state for weight loss and management. Keep the glycemic index of your foods as low as possible.

3. Complex carbohydrates should be preferred over simple carbohydrates.

4. Decrease saturated fats. Use blood type–appropriate monounsaturated and polyunsaturated fats instead.

5. Eat a minimum of one to three large servings of dark leafy vegetables (such as kale, chard, collard greens, mustard greens, dandelion greens, or arugula) each day. The variety will depend upon your blood type requirements.

6. Eat unprocessed foods whenever possible. Choose fresh foods.

7. Eat organic foods whenever possible.

8. Drink plenty of water (alkaline).

# Dietary Analysis

Please list ALL the foods and liquids that you consume for three days—*including the amounts*. **Important:** Remember to include ALL the "Avoid" foods and junk foods such as Oreos, slices of pizza, cans of soda, etc.

## Day 1:

Breakfast _____

Midmorning _____

Noon _____

Midafternoon _____

Dinner _____

After dinner _____

## Day 2:

Breakfast _____

Midmorning _____

Noon _____

Midafternoon _____

Dinner _____

After dinner _____

## Day 3:

Breakfast _____

Midmorning _____

Noon _____

Midafternoon _____

Dinner _____

After dinner _____

If you take nutritional supplements, please list them:

_____

_____

_____

# Chapter 3

# BLOOD TYPE AND WEIGHT LOSS

I N SECTION II of this book I will be addressing the issue of how you can become an "instinctive eater" as it applies to the blood-type diet theory. I will teach you the basics of why and what to eat for the rest of your life to improve your health and illness profile, and specifically how instinctive eating is the basis for reaching your ideal weight for life.

Before I take you there, however, I want to focus on your goals for losing weight and the role your blood type plays in this effort. You will notice as you read this chapter that I make reference to the thermogenic weight-loss program instead of the blood-type weight-loss diet. The reason is simply because of how my fat-burning meal replacements, when working in concert with the blood-type diet concept, create a thermogenic or fat-burning effect in the body—the perfect combination for jump-starting your metabolism. But when your expectations for losing weight and keeping it off for life are high, the anticipation of that reality can be devastating if you do not reach your goals, particularly if you are stuck in the old mentality of "dieting" your weight off. From this point forward, you will see that there is a much more effective and simpler approach to this weight-loss issue than you ever thought.

## KEEPING WEIGHT LOSS SIMPLE

My approach to weight loss and keeping it off for life is based on your body mechanics and bodily functions as the key elements for losing weight successfully. It is simple to be successful at losing weight and keeping it off for life if you remember to apply these two basic principles:

1. Jump-start your metabolism; then feed it to keep it in motion.

2. Eat food compatible to your blood type, and don't diet.

When you begin to understand the vital role that bodily functions (metabolism) play in losing weight, you will soon discover that all the efforts you have used through sheer willpower to "hang in there" with diets have become a thing of the past. My approach for losing weight will minimize your effort and maximize the results by allowing your body to be the "natural" calorie burner it was designed to be.

### Your attitude

To be successful, you must first be willing to *change*, which starts with a change in your mental attitude. Though this attitude change is one of the toughest exercises you and I face, it is fundamental for success.

As you think about the various areas in your life that can interfere with your ability to lose weight or maintain proper weight afterward, you will agree that a *change of attitude* plays an absolutely huge part in your success or failure. The way you think about yourself directly affects the success or failure toward losing weight.

For example, people who struggle with their weight sometimes have poor self-image issues or lack self-value or worth. This may be due to a number of emotional factors that had to do with their upbringing but ultimately manifest themselves in eating behaviorisms. These emotional triggers can cause the individual to self-medicate with food in hopes of solving the emotional issue they are dealing with and thereby interfering with a healthy attitude toward eating. In addition, when these emotional issues are unresolved, they tend to be the underlying root cause to backsliding once you have lost the weight. Other people find themselves suffering from being overweight because of poor eating habits such as eating on the run, late-night snacking, or improper food selections. They need to change the way they think about eating. Nearly every client I have had has said that they lack the time to eat proper meals—especially breakfast—because of hectic schedules. Many people say they do not have time for exercise. The lack of regular exercise contributes to failure to lose weight, so if a person needs to lose weight, he or she needs to think differently about making exercise a part of their lifestyle.

Some don't know what to think about their weight problem, so they just try various protocols, hoping something good will happen. Those who take medications with side effects that prohibit weight loss or cause weight gain will need to refocus their attention on eradicating the root problem so they can in turn reduce or eliminate the use of medications (if applicable).

In the end, your success for losing weight and keeping it off for life will depend to a large extent on your willingness to make necessary changes such as those mentioned above. It will also involve analyzing your current state of health, your lifestyle, and your level of determination and desire to win the battle.

## Your metabolism

Now, there is one more thing. We must address the issue of your body's mechanics or bodily functions. These are the keys to successful weight loss and keeping it off for life. These keys unlock the secret of your *metabolism*. Before you can expect to lose your first pound, you have to learn to ignite or stimulate your metabolism and then keep it in perpetual motion. Once you get your metabolism in motion, the weight-loss process begins automatically because you are in the process of improving your BMR (basal metabolic rate).

The BMR, which reflects your body's ability to burn calories while you are resting, is the key to understanding your body as a calorie-burning machine. Regardless of how much weight you need to lose or how quickly you want to lose it, improving your body's basal metabolic rate is the key to your success.

Think for a moment about how many hours a day you are *inactive*—sitting, lying down, sleeping—versus the hours you are *active*, and you begin to understand your need to rev up that BMR. Therefore, your primary focal point for weight loss must be on ways to stimulate your metabolism. This focus will keep your mind thinking correctly and will help to deter it from rethinking former thoughts related to "dieting." Results from the calorie-burning effect that come from stimulating your metabolism are far greater and longer lasting than you could ever expect from "dieting it off." The two most effective methods for stimulating your metabolism are *eating* and *exercising*. For now, we will focus on eating.

## THE "FIRE" IN YOUR FIREPLACE

Let me give you a simple picture story or analogy to help you get a handle on weight loss for life. The story draws a parallel between your body's ability to burn calories and the way a fire in your fireplace warms your family room. The fire is symbolic of your metabolism; the kindling or wood that is burned by the fire is symbolic of food calories your metabolism burns. The end result, a warm family room from the blazing fire in your fireplace, is symbolic of you reaching your weight-loss goals for life by keeping your metabolism in perpetual motion.

Since I am originally from Buffalo, New York, where the winter weather is extremely cold, I can easily relate to the pleasure and enjoyment (not to mention the necessity) of a blazing fire in the fireplace. Try to imagine that you are living in Buffalo, New York, in the middle of winter—high temperatures do not climb above 20 degrees, and the frigid lows plummet to below zero.

If you plan to survive such a winter by warming the family room where you spend most of your time indoors, then knowing how to make a fire in the fireplace that will burn continually is vitally important. Your goal is to keep the family room warm day and night. To achieve your goal, you will need to know first how to ignite the fire and, second, how to *sustain* it indefinitely to maintain its heating capacity.

### Igniting the fire

You will need special combustible materials like kindling to ignite a fire in your family room fireplace. By igniting the kindling you create a flame, which is capable of burning more kindling. It is also important to choose dry kindling to readily ignite a fire and avoid excessive smoke. Obviously, the flame created by kindling is not powerful enough to warm the family room, but it is a start. To get the blazing fire you need for warmth, all you need to do is add more kindling—regularly—along with larger-sized logs. As the fire blazes, it burns the kindling easily, which ignites the logs, and your expectation of having a warm family room becomes a reality.

### Sustaining the fire

Since a warm family room is dependent on the warmth generated by the fire, the second step to insure that warmth is to keep the fire burning. Maintaining the fire is easier than igniting the fire because all you have to do to keep the family room warm is to continue to *feed the fire*. It is important to realize that should you stop feeding the fire, it will go out, and the room will grow cold again. If that happens, you will have to start the entire process over again by igniting the kindling.

### Applying the "fire" analogy

The parallel between the blazing fire in the family room, which easily burns the kindling, is the manner in which your metabolism will burn calories if it remains *stimulated*. Using the right kind of kindling is important for igniting the fire, and adding logs keeps the fire blazing for comfortable warmth. In that same way, foods you eat that are compatible to your blood type are necessary to keeping your metabolism "burning" more efficiently. The faster the metabolic rate, the easier it is for your body to burn calories. And the longer you eat this way for sustaining your metabolism, the easier it will be to reach and maintain your ideal weight for life.

## Thermogenesis: Igniting Your Body's Fire

To get from our analogy of igniting and sustaining the fire in the fireplace to the specifics of achieving your weight-loss goals, we need to consider two parallel steps: *thermogenesis* and *metabolic momentum*.

The first step to take before you can expect to lose weight is to "ignite" or *stimulate* your metabolism. Just like igniting the fire in the fireplace, you must ignite your metabolism through a process called thermogenesis. Thermogenesis allows the body to burn fat to create energy.

For thermogenesis to occur, you must create a thermodynamic effect in the body by stimulating specific fat-cell receptors, which will then elicit a breakdown of fat. This process for breaking down stored fat is known as *lipolysis*. Lipolysis causes the body to use stored fat as fuel for energy. Simultaneously, this stimulation causes an increase in your metabolic rate and is the precursor for creating *metabolic momentum*. By increasing your metabolic rate, your body becomes that "natural" fat burner it was designed to be, and you begin losing weight.

### Metabolic momentum

Just like feeding more logs to the blazing fire in your fireplace throughout the day, you can create metabolic momentum by feeding your body, which stimulates your metabolism. Metabolic momentum, like thermodynamics, creates a perpetual state of internal energy production or calorie burning, which is imperative for weight loss. If kept up long enough, maintaining your metabolic momentum will cause you to reach your ideal weight and maintain it for life. Imagine! The most natural and sensible way to keep your metabolism in perpetual motion is by *eating*—not by depriving yourself of food through dieting! And making the right food selections compatible to your blood type is extremely effective for igniting your metabolic momentum, much like selecting dry kindling to ignite a clean fire readily.

## Why eat foods compatible to your blood type?

Have you ever tried to ignite a fire with wet twigs? It is a difficult task and one that results in more acrid smoke than actual flame. Eating foods that are not compatible to your blood type is like trying to ignite a fire with wet twigs. As you discover the many benefits you will receive by making food selections compatible to your blood type (A), you will see how certain foods actually cause you to gain or lose weight. Keep in mind that this approach is not generic but individualized based on your genetics. When I struggled for over ten years with hypoglycemia, I ate very little red meat but more carbohydrates from pastas, breads, and so on. Once I realized what I was doing to my bodily systems and functions, and started eating foods compatible to my blood type, not only did my blood sugar stabilize, but also I started dropping body fat. Adding compatible vegetables like broccoli and kale in my salads and eating foods that were compatible helped my metabolism become a raging fire. As you make food selections (kindling) that are compatible to your blood type, your body will burn calories more efficiently because the protein molecules (lectins) found in these foods do not interfere with proper digestion and assimilation of calories.

In fact, eating compatible food for your blood type assists the body in losing weight by eliminating excess toxins that are stored in the fat cells, which in turn shrinks the size of your fat cells. Selecting food that is compatible to your blood type also serves as a medicine for healing and repairing bodily functions, which is absolutely necessary for calorie expenditure.

### Why avoid incompatible foods?

Foods that are incompatible for your blood type will slow down your metabolic rate, making it difficult to lose weight and possibly even causing weight gain.

As a blood type A individual, you are unique and will see how this genetically based approach to making food selections is most crucial to your success in reaching your ideal weight for life. Being a type A, you will discover, besides the guidelines I have stated previously, your success will lie in choosing the right foods and avoiding the wrong foods to lose weight and maintain it. For example, heavy proteins like red meat will store as fat, cause increase in digestive toxins, and digest poorly, all leading to weight gain. Take one more example—dairy. Dairy foods will disrupt proper nutrient utilization. This is why I listed the beneficial, neutral, and avoid food group categories for you in the book so you can successfully reach your ideal weight loss/gain goals for life by being accurate.

Dietary lectins are another food component that can work for you or against you as you seek to reach your weight goals, depending on whether the food is compatible with your particular blood type. When a food with a dietary lectin is beneficial for you, it is because the lectins function as scavengers that remove debris and toxins from various systems in the body—liver, blood, intestines, and so forth.

Foods with dietary lectins that work *against* your normal bodily functions are considered "avoid" foods (not junk foods), and you need to stay away from them. Let's use wheat as an example of an avoid food since it is very common. Wheat—whether whole wheat or refined wheat—has wheat gluten agglutinin lectin (found in the kernel), which makes it incompatible for most people. As the wheat product is digested, the lectins attach or glue themselves to the red blood cells in the gut wall, creating a clumping of cells, known as agglutination. This clumping effect breaks down the function of that particular system and, in this case, interferes with proper digestion. Since the body is sensitive and very responsive, it sends out signals or symptoms like gas, bloating, or worse—such as IBS or colon inflammation—indicating that something is wrong. Until that particular food is avoided, that system cannot heal or return to normal function, regardless of ways we choose to medicate the symptoms.

Agglutination occurs in any system in the body. For example, if the insulin cell receptors are affected by a particular food that is not compatible, it will *slow* down the metabolic process and cause the body to store calories—exactly the opposite of what you want to happen. So by virtue of avoiding foods with dietary lectins that work against the bodily systems for certain blood types, the body can return to normal function and induce optimum health and metabolic function.

A maximum metabolic rate can be produced by eating food that is compatible to your blood type and avoiding food that is not. It's the biochemical response to food compatible with your blood type that promotes ideal weight for life. As your body responds favorably by eating according to your blood type, the results are improved bodily and systemic function. As I mentioned earlier, my approach to losing weight has everything to do with our bodily functions or mechanics. For our purpose, selecting foods that are compatible for your blood type (red blood cells) improves the body's digestive and metabolic systems, which means a faster metabolism (blazing fire), better nutrient assimilation, and digestion.

Everyone must eat to survive, so why not eat the foods best suited for you?

## RECAP

Losing weight and reaching your ideal weight for life has never been so easy yet so misunderstood—until now! Simply remember the following:

1. *Thermogenesis* is the igniting and stimulating effect on your metabolism and is responsible for starting the calorie-burning process. Thermogenesis also serves as a precursor for creating metabolic momentum.

2. *Metabolic momentum* is keeping your metabolism in perpetual motion.

3. *Eating* is one of the most efficient methods for maintaining metabolic momentum—not food deprivation through dieting.

4. Eating food that is *compatible to your blood type* is an individualized method of eating for obtaining maximum health, reducing illness, losing weight, and maintaining your ideal weight for life.

Chapter 4

# TYPE A: EVERYTHING
# YOU NEED TO KNOW

A S MAN MIGRATED geographically to locations where meat was not readily available, environmental adaptation was required for survival, which involved adaptation to a different diet—specifically vegetarian. These early migrations were to places like Europe, Asia, and Australia, regions totally different from the plentiful plains of Africa where animal protein was abundant. These early migrators learned to survive on fruits, vegetables, and grains. As a result, many people with blood type A do best avoiding almost all animal protein in favor of a vegetarian diet.

Individuals with type A blood have the thickest blood of all blood types. In the United States, meat and potatoes have comprised the traditional staple diet. Type As do not tolerate either meat or potatoes well. When type As eat these foods that are inconsistent with their blood type, their already thick blood agglutinates, or gets thicker and stickier. The thick blood requires the heart to pump harder, inevitably causing high blood pressure, hypertension, an enlarged heart muscle, and an increase in heart disease. This is the major reason why type A individuals have the shortest life span today.

Another downside for individuals with type A blood is that in their adaptation to a vegetarian diet, over time type As began to secrete less stomach acid necessary to metabolize meat protein. Type As have very low stomach acid by genetic standards; while the low acid accommodates the metabolism of fruits and vegetables, it does a miserable job metabolizing animal protein.

A constant diet of mainly meats and potatoes provides fewer nutrients to the body, lowers immune function, and thickens the blood, leading to heart disease, cancer, and earlier death. For precisely these reasons, type As are susceptible to heart disease and cancer. The Japanese are an exception; they eat a staple diet of fish, rice, and green tea—the perfect diet for individuals of type A blood.[1]

*Strengths:*

- Adapts well to dietary and environmental changes

*Weaknesses:*

- Thick blood

- Shortest life span

- Affected by stress more than other blood groups

- Sensitive digestive tract

- Vulnerable immune system

- Must avoid almost all animal protein

*Health risks:*

- Heart disease

- Cancer

- High blood pressure and hypertension

- Enlarged heart muscle

- Decreased immune function

- Anemia

- Liver disorders

- Gallbladder disorders

- Diabetes

*Nutritional profile:*

- Eat soybeans and tofu, and drink green tea for antioxidant qualities; eat grouper, cod, and salmon; eat soy cheese and drink soy milk; eat lentils, broccoli, carrots, romaine lettuce, spinach, blueberries, blackberries, cranberries, prunes, raisins

- Avoid animal fat; meat or dairy products; meat-and-potato diet; kidney, lima, and navy beans; durum wheat; eggplant; peppers; tomatoes; cantaloupe; honeydew melons

In my book *The Answer Is in Your Bloodtype*, a composite study of disease and mortality statistics conducted with approximately 5,200 individuals based on gender, age, blood type, and disease is analyzed. What we found were some very interesting statistics and conclusions. For example, it was the blood type A (and AB because of the dominant A gene) that showed the greatest potential for heart disease, such as heart attack or heart failure, and cancer to occur prematurely or earlier than the other blood types. It appeared that the other blood types seemed to have dodged the bullet, so to speak, and not experience similar illnesses until later in life. We came to the conclusion that with all things being normal, these diseases or illnesses were lifestyle related and therefore could be prevented or eliminated by lifestyle changes—eating accurately for one's blood type!

The foods most harmful to As in the long run are meat and dairy. The elimination of these two food groups will allow type A individuals the greatest potential to avoid heart disease and cancer. Tofu, soy products, unsalted redskin peanuts, red wine, and green tea are especially good for type As because they help fight cancer.[2] Type As typically have lost the ability to make pepsin, a protein-digesting enzyme. Therefore, a more vegetarian diet, or one of less-dense protein products such as chicken, turkey, and Cornish hens, is more easily digestible for As. Whole grains such as quinoa, millet, brown rice, and wild rice are preferable over wheat products due to oversensitivity to such products.[3]

Listen to your body. If what you are eating does not agree with you, *stop*.

## POSITIONED FOR SUCCESS

As you have learned throughout this section, your genetics have determined what you are and how your body responds, reacts, and performs. With the understanding of the principles I have outlined in these first four chapters, you are positioned for success—just as soon as you get started. By applying the information and strategies set forth in this book, you will discover how to eat foods compatible to your blood type.

Genetically speaking, you and I have been given just so much clay to work with. Why not follow the right path and enjoy the journey reaching your genetic potential?

My desire is to help you reach a new level of improved health, physical appearance, and an energetic life as quickly as possible. But please remember, it is your *journey in life* that is most important. Your genetic predisposition is basic to your success. As you better understand the role your genetics play, you will better understand the science behind the dietary strategies through this book.

As your journey continues to section II of this book, take what you have learned, appropriate the experiences you have applied to your lifestyle, and pass them along for the good of others. That will add more worth to your life. *Roads were not built for destinations—they were built for the journey.*

## RECAP

There are specific characteristics of each blood type in relation to nutrition. Since you are type A, simply remember the following:

1. The two primary food groups you need to avoid for the long haul are meat and dairy. Your inability to properly digest and assimilate these food groups, particularly meats, will contribute to worsening your illness profile and interfering with you reaching and maintaining your ideal weight for life.

2. Your protein sources should be vegetarian-like, but less-dense protein from turkey, chicken, and even Cornish hen will work fine.

3. Minimum wheat will work OK in your diet, but your oversensitivity to it will stir up sinus issues and perhaps asthmatic-like symptoms as well, so be very conservative with wheat.

4. Drink a glass of water with lemon every morning upon rising. Due to your naturally sensitive tissue, you have more mucus in your airway membranes that acts as a safeguard against tissue inflammation. The acid of lemon will cut the mucus buildup that you have in the mornings.

# SECTION II

# THE BLOOD TYPE
# EATING PLAN

# Chapter 5

# HOW TO BECOME AN INSTINCTIVE EATER

INSTINCTIVE EATING IS uniquely different from the typical diet plan. Instinctive eating requires that you grasp hold of your genetic or cellular profile, using that knowledge as the baseline or fundamental foundation for the way you eat.

You will understand the difference between diet plans and instinctive eating as you read the following pages. But more important than what you read—*you will experience the difference once you give it your best shot.* My intention here is to help you see what instinctive eating is and why it makes good sense to implement it as a part of your lifestyle. So if you are a dieter, have tried dieting to some degree, or would like to take your first healthy step in the right direction, then get ready for some fascinating and life-changing information that you can try for yourself.

My experience throughout the years has taught me that the greatest majority of people who have searched for a diet plan wanted one that would help them to reach a goal of permanent weight loss. Yet seldom—if ever—have they found a plan that could succeed at that! For one reason or another, the plan they chose did not work—at least not for permanent weight loss. No doubt the main reason was that it was just too difficult to adapt to that diet plan as a lifestyle change.

Most people would love to find the answer to their fatigue, weight, and health problems so they could feel better and enjoy their lives more. That's a normal human desire. But sometimes it takes a wake-up call to get a person's attention—something like a heart attack, stomach disorder, or chronic illness that steals your money and, more importantly, your life.

The desire to better ourselves and to live longer is within each of us. It's part of our natural, innate mechanism for survival. My main objectives are to get you on the path to instinctive eating and to keep you from the frustrating and unnecessary physical and emotional roller-coaster rides so often associated with diets.

If you have sought long-term results by following a diet plan that focuses strictly on end results, now would be a great time to take your first step by changing your thinking. Just the thought of going on a diet causes words to surface, words like *sacrifice, deprivation, going without,* and *struggling to stay on a diet.*

Who said that making healthier food selections was a matter of pure sacrifice? Who said you could never deviate from the letter of the law? Certainly not me! That kind of behavioral response has caused thousands of people like yourself to end up thinking that making healthy food selections is nothing more than a punishment/reward system of eating. Consequently, this mind-set will prohibit lifestyle adaptation.

The problem with this diet mentality is this: the focus is on the end results. It disregards the essentials—improving your health, becoming disease free, and living a longer, healthier life with more energy. These essentials require a lifestyle adaptation.

You may have been victimized by the commercial slants placing all the emphasis on cosmetic results—not lifestyle. If you are wondering if marketing the "body beautiful" is a powerful tool, just ask any marketing genius from one of the huge weight-loss companies. I am sure they will tell you that it is much harder to sell good health than it is to sell the promise of beauty. Understand what I am saying here. While each one of us will have motivational influences that initially engage us to make dietary changes, in order to be successful over the long haul we must focus on the journey—not the destination.

## FOCUS ON THE JOURNEY

The road you travel, the path you choose to enjoy the journey of your life, needs to become your focus point, not merely the destination. When the focus is placed on the wrong thing, failure is inevitable. That is why the majority of the diet plans you have tried before never lasted.

As you analyze your dieting experiences in retrospect, you will probably agree that they were more of a "suck-it-up-and-give-it-all-the-willpower-you-can-muster-for-as-long-as-you-can" kind of experience—definitely not a journey.

Focusing on the journey offers many more rewards along the way than focusing only on the end results. The journey experience allows you to enjoy the many benefits available by making adaptable dietary changes for a lifetime. These benefits come in many packages.

> ### Benefits of the Journey Experience
> ❑ Continual awareness of your body's reactions to certain foods
> ❑ Realization of the positive or negative side effects from certain foods
> ❑ A constant increase in energy
> ❑ Better cholesterol readings
> ❑ Less need for medications
> ❑ Less down time caused by sickness and ill health

Focusing on the journey will help you to enjoy life by spending more time with your family and friends and less time visiting hospitals and doctors. The path or road you decide to travel determines the lifestyle with which you will live.

Are you ready to make your choice? Are you ready to begin the journey?

## INSTINCTIVE EATING

In chapter 3, I outlined the weight-loss principles to follow if losing weight is your goal. I also mentioned that the primary purpose for those steps is to help jump-start your metabolism so you can lose weight. And ultimately, this plan will teach you that *eating* instead of *dieting* is the healthy and natural way to be successful with your weight and health for life. So in this section of the book you will learn how to become an instinctive eater. You may be asking the question: What is an instinctive eater? Instinctive eating is best understood by observing the creatures in the animal kingdom.

Let's look at the lioness as one example. This cool cat has never taken a course in Nutrition 101 or purchased the latest weight-loss diet plan on the market. She was never influenced by medical and scientific documentation teaching her that all food is OK to eat as long as she ate it in moderation. This feline has never been formally educated.

But how fascinating it is to note that the lioness possesses something far superior to what has—or has not been—scientifically proven. She has a dietary mechanism for survival, which is *instinctive eating.* When it comes to eating, there are no guidelines for her to follow. There are no daily menus to follow. But when dinnertime rolls around, she absolutely knows what she should eat. The lioness will always order meat for dinner. She would not be caught dead climbing a banana tree to eat bananas.

Her eating habits are not accidental. Nor are they coincidental. Animals eat instinctively because their inherent, natural dietary mechanism for survival determines what they eat.

Consider the horse for a moment. A horse is a horse, of course. But when was the last time you saw a farmer strap a feed bag filled with chopped beef onto a horse? Try going to your local 4-H club to ask if chopped beef is OK for your horse. You would be laughed out of the barn. A horse's feed bag is always filled with oats.

Put a horse out to pasture, and it will naturally eat grass. Did you ever see a horse run through a pasture chasing squirrels or rabbits for a midafternoon snack?

You would be intrigued by what you can learn about animals. For example, did you know that most animals of the same species generally live to be the same age? Their dietary mechanism for survival allows them to live to the potential life span of that species. A very few may die of cancer or other rare diseases or get killed by a predator, but most animals die of old age.

Not so for us humanoids; we are different. We generally die at a young age from a variety of different diseases, many of which are associated with our diets. Or we live out our last years in a less-than-desirable physical condition. I have always said that when it is my turn to go to heaven, I want to check out of Dodge City doing 180 miles per hour—not spending the last twenty years of life using a walker because I was negligent with my health.

The very thought of living to be one hundred years of age is, for most humans, quite a stretch. Up until now we did not have a clue about how to eat instinctively. Most people eat for reasons that fall far short of supplying our bodies with sound nutrition, good health, and longevity. We all come from a huge dietary mixing bowl that swings like a pendulum. Some people or groups insist that everybody should be a vegetarian, while others refuse to give up their meats. Others will support the high-carbohydrate, zero-protein-and-fat diet, while others support a high-protein, high-fat, and no-carbohydrate diet. Throw in our taste buds, ethnic traditions, religious beliefs, social settings, and the dilemma of the emotional, bulimic, or anorexic eater, and it is easy to see why we have a lot to learn from the dietary instincts of our "inferior" animal counterparts.

Unless you have lived with gorillas for many years and learned all about instinctive eating as Anthony Hopkins did in the movie *Instinct*, how could you experience benefits from instinctive eating? How could you become an instinctive eater if at first you didn't have some guidelines or dietary strategies from which to learn? Remember, we have never been enlightened to know how to eat instinctively. We must first learn.

The dietary guidelines in this book are based on blood type A. I believe personally that I am communicating to you an approach to eating that is the most effective, individual, and accurate method of making food selections that can become an adaptable lifestyle change. Because this method is genetically based, it will prove itself by the many ways your body responds to certain foods.

I do not expect you to take my word for it without some basic understanding and ultimately testing its validity for yourself. This is especially true when it comes to making dietary changes. The dietary changes must not impose restrictions so unrealistic that you find it impossible to reach your goals or so unattainable that the changes cannot become part of your lifestyle.

On the other hand, you must remember that anything worth doing is worth doing right. My desire is to help you live a healthy, more energetic, and sickness-free life for as long as possible. What I am recommending is doable. If it wasn't realistic enough to live with, we would both be wasting our time. I want you to become a "believer" like me and thousands of others who have put this dietary approach to the test.

## GENETIC BASELINE

I mentioned briefly in chapter 1 that one of the primary reasons why different blood types respond differently to certain foods is due to the effect dietary lectins have on your body. I'd like to explain how this works in more detail now, because it relates to the instinctive approach to eating.

Dietary lectins are protein molecules found in food. If a food is not compatible to your blood type, these lectins can create havoc in your body systems. These negative responses occur due to a chemical phenomenon referred to as *agglutination*. The lectins will bond themselves randomly to blood cells in an organ or bodily system and begin to interfere with the natural and normal function of that particular system or organ.

Typically, blood cells have a slippery surface and are unaffected by dietary lectins as long as the host consumes foods that are compatible. But dietary lectins present in foods that are incompatible with your blood type wreak havoc by attaching themselves to the blood cell.

Think for a moment about what would happen if you tried to roll a tennis ball over a strip of Velcro. The tennis ball would stick to that Velcro strip just like glue and be impossible to roll. This is what happens when you ingest foods that are not compatible to your blood type. Instead of the dietary lectins rolling over the blood cells in that system, they will stick like glue to the surface of the blood cells.

Let's take your digestive system for example. Suppose you consume some food that is not compatible to your blood type. The dietary lectins begin to attach themselves to the blood cells on the wall of your intestines. As this process continues, a clumping of blood cells takes place that begins to interfere with the normal function of that digestive system. Now your problems have just begun.

You may not be aware this is taking place, but your digestive system knows. It just took a hit, and it is beginning its downward spiral. Your body knows that it has just been poisoned, and it tries to let you know by sending you signals or warning signs. Sometimes these warnings or signals are subtle and less dangerous, giving you symptoms like gas, bloating, or indigestion, things we normally just ignore.

But ignoring these symptoms is a dangerous thing to do. They often indicate a serious problem or disease that needs an immediate solution if we want to maintain good health.

If these symptoms persist, the next order of business is usually to medicate. Medicating a symptom is a behavioral reaction that most people do when they discover that part of their normal bodily function is malfunctioning. They respond this way because of their immediate need for satisfaction and relief. Often they are also unaware of good prevention and cure techniques.

Instead of addressing the root problem that is causing your body to send out these helpful warnings to you, you end up experiencing the possible loss of function of that system by medicating the symptoms. The time finally comes when these warnings can no longer be ignored or sufficiently medicated. You become nearly incapacitated by cramping, abdominal pain, continual fatigue, and the lack of energy.

Soon you find yourself dealing with chronic digestive disorders like diverticulitis, irritable bowel syndrome (IBS), celiac disease, and possibly the eventuality of cancer of the colon. At this point, your quality of life has taken a major dive.

How unfortunate it would be if your house was on fire and the firemen came and squirted water only on the smoke. With that kind of negligent approach, it would not be very long before there was nothing left of your home. This is exactly what happens to your health and quality of life when you ignore the warning signs that your body is sending out.

Instinctive eating can help you to pick up immediately on the signals your body is sending. You will quickly become aware of the negative responses your body warns you about when you eat incompatible foods.

The things that I just described about your digestive system do not have to happen to your health. You can avoid them by learning to become an instinctive eater. You only have one body to carry you throughout life; why wouldn't you want to take care of it?

One day as I was mailing books at the local post office, one of the clerks asked me what the book was all about. After explaining the concept to her, I asked her why she had asked.

She told me that she had constant stomach pain and was taking medication for it. She was overweight and tired all the time. I gave her a book and told her to follow the dietary guidelines and menus for at least three weeks. I advised her to do her best to avoid the avoid foods listed for her blood type.

As we talked, I asked her if she was a blood type B, which she said she was. I told her it would be imperative to avoid eating chicken. She was flabbergasted, because chicken was her staple. She ate it almost daily.

About three weeks later I went back to the post office, and out from behind the counter this woman jumped. "What do you think?" she asked. (Keep in mind that I didn't know her.) Before I could say anything, she said that she had dropped sixteen pounds. She had no more stomach pain, was off her medications, and felt great. Plus, she had tons of energy.

She confessed that one day her daughter brought over some fried chicken, but she ate only one piece. Twenty-four hours after she ate it, she had an upset stomach. The taste of the chicken had actually been totally unappealing to her. "I never would have believed it if I didn't try it," she said to me. "It was the easiest thing I ever did!"

Learning to be an instinctive eater may not be the easiest thing you will ever learn to do—but it will be one of the healthiest things you ever do for yourself. The next chapter will help you to get started by showing you how to complete a simple four-week test for instinctive eating. It's one test you will be glad you took.

## RECAP

Simply remember the following:

1. View this approach to eating as a lifestyle not like going on a restrictive diet.

2. Follow the guidelines I have set forth in the book for your blood type.

3. Test what I am teaching you, and your body will confirm it to be true.

4. Become an instinctive eater. Listen to your body. Your body is the best teacher.

# Chapter 6

# GETTING STARTED:
# THE FOUR-WEEK TEST

NOW THAT YOU have had an informal crash course in Instinctive Eating 101, you have a better understanding about the connection that exists between your specific blood type and the food you eat. By now you should be motivated to test this concept and prove it for yourself.

This four-week test period is what I refer to as your window of opportunity. If you will take this opportunity, believing that your good health is worth this investment of time, I believe you will discover for yourself that what I have told you will work for you.

This information can become your ticket to great health. By following the dietary and exercise guidelines in this book, you can turn your health around, control your weight, increase your energy, stabilize your blood sugar, lower your cholesterol and blood pressure, and possibly get off prescription medications once and for all.

Our Creator did not make any mistakes when He made you and me. He created us to live long, healthy lives, and He placed on this earth all the necessary food sources for us to do just that. Just because we may not understand something new or unfamiliar does not mean we should discard it as useless to us.

The world of science is making continual biological advancements. Science is decoding and breaking down the understanding of DNA codes at a surprising rate. An entirely new world of health possibilities is right around the corner. Daily we are learning to better understand our bodies and how to keep them in optimal health.

Learning how to more accurately appropriate these new discoveries and biological findings may one day show us how to prevent diseases before they occur, simply by addressing the root issues. Something as simple as adapting to a better dietary lifestyle by making behavior changes in advance of the onset of disease instead of after disease invades our body can increase our potential for living longer and healthier.

This simple four-week test will give you the opportunity to experience for yourself, without any outside influences, that what I am telling you is real—and that it works. It will answer many of your questions about whether there truly is a connection or link between your blood type and diet, health, disease, energy, weight loss, low blood sugar, sugar cravings, and longevity. Keep in mind that individual results will vary because we are all different, even those of the same blood type. Each person is still uniquely made. Because none of us share the same physical conditions, medical history, or body genetics, it is imperative for you to let your body be your only teacher. You can do that as you learn to become an instinctive eater.

## BEGINNING YOUR FOUR-WEEK TEST

Check with your physician before you begin your four-week test and before following these dietary guidelines. This four-week test is not to be misconstrued as a substitute for medical recommendations.

For the next four weeks, you will be monitoring the foods you eat. You will choose from the food groupings given in this book. However, the important thing to remember will be to choose from the appropriate food groupings for you. There are approximately sixteen food groups given, which include all the various foods we eat as well as condiments, spices, and juices. These food groups will give you a wonderful array of food to choose from, with many varieties in each group.

There are three categories for each food group—beneficial foods, neutral foods, and avoid foods:

1. Beneficial foods—foods that your body, according to your blood type, treats as medicine for healing systems and improving bodily function and performance

2. Neutral foods—foods that your body, according to your blood type, treats as compatible sources of energy

3. Avoid foods—foods that your body, according to your blood type, treats as poisons and toxins. (These are not junk food. They may be your favorite food, one all this time you thought was good for you.)

## Window of Opportunity

The four-week test can be your window of opportunity. To get the most accurate results, follow the guidelines given below.

### Avoid the avoid foods

During the next four weeks, do your best to avoid eating the avoid foods listed for your blood type. No one will be 100 percent successful at doing this, but give it your best attempt. Look for continued progress—not perfection. Avoid foods are foods that are not compatible with your specific blood type; therefore, they should be avoided.

During this test period your body will undergo a detoxification process. Much of the detoxifying will take place within your digestive system, which is greatly influenced by the association of your blood type and dietary lectins from the food you eat. You will begin experiencing some wonderful changes. Some of the symptoms that you may have been experiencing prior to this test, such as gas, bloating, irritable bowel syndrome, and gastroesophageal reflux disorder (GERD), have been known to disappear during this test period. In most cases, these symptoms disappear in just a few days.

Within weeks, you may also experience a considerable drop in your elevated cholesterol and blood pressure levels—without the use of medications. If you struggle with hypoglycemia, or low blood sugar, your blood sugar levels will stabilize.

Within several days, you could discover that you have more than enough energy to last all day long instead of feeling your energy drop off in the middle of the day, as I did while struggling with hypoglycemia for fifteen long, unbearable years.

Thank Yahweh, I haven't had low blood sugar problems since.

Along with the foods you avoid, avoid also the diet mentality that focuses on the end results only. Do not become trapped by thoughts of what you cannot eat. That's the old way of diet thinking. The avoidance of the avoid foods is not a form of punishment, nor is it a form of imprisonment. You can eat anything you want! But by adhering to these guidelines for this test period, you will have the opportunity to experience a cleansing and relief from some of the digestive disorders your body has been dealing with.

Keep in mind that the avoid foods play havoc with blood lipids and the proper function of your digestive system, immune system, liver, and kidneys. The more you adhere to the guidelines for the test period, the greater the opportunity for your body to rid itself of damaging dietary lectins. Eliminating these dietary lectins found in the avoid foods will give you positive results now—and long term. You will accumulate the knowledge you need to truly become an instinctive eater.

Avoiding the avoid foods for your blood type will bring another benefit—weight loss! The toxins that have been stored up in the fat cells of your body as a result of eating the wrong foods will be eliminated, and the fat cells will begin to shrink as part of the detoxification process. Your digestive system and your metabolism will start to function properly and more efficiently as you eliminate dietary lectins, like wheat gluten, that slow down metabolism and digestive system functions. The results will be a healthy colon, a speedy metabolism, and loss in body fat—all without going on a diet! I refer to the loss of body fat as a by-product of instinctive eating—not the by-product of dieting. I think you will agree.

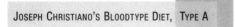

## Concentrate on the beneficial foods

You may be wondering, "If I avoid the avoid foods, what can I find to eat?" You will have a delectable array of good nutritious foods from which to choose. Simply make your food selections from the fourteen-day menus, or pick and choose your favorite food selections from the beneficial foods category for your blood type.

As you consider your food choices, you will discover that there are more food selections in the beneficial foods and neutral foods than you found on the avoid foods list, so don't despair. Do not even bother trying to count calories during the four-week test period—just eat. A good rule to follow is this: eat when you are hungry, but stop when you are comfortably satisfied.

In some of the food groupings, you will see that there are no beneficial foods from which to choose. Your first choice should be to forgo that particular food group, but if you must make a selection, do so from the neutral foods. Remember, the more correctly you eat for your blood type, the better the results, and your beneficial foods will promote the best results.

Once you complete the test period, your body has experienced a thorough cleansing and overhaul. You should have some wonderful experiences to share. Many people have called, e-mailed, or written my office to share their positive experiences during their four-week test. I would love to hear from you too. (See page 165 for contact information.)

## Monitor your progress

It will be important to monitor your responses during this four-week period. Here are four important steps in the monitoring process:

1. If possible, have blood work done to know your current cholesterol readings before you start.

2. If possible, have your blood pressure taken before you start.

3. Record medication dosages, which medications, and for what condition you are taking them.

4. Record your progress using the chart on page 72.

As you learn to eat correctly for your blood type, your body will function more properly, your metabolism will stay revved up, and your digestive system will operate more efficiently. You will be able to control your weight without dieting and live longer with less to no incapacitating illnesses. More importantly, you will be able to enjoy your life to its fullest.

Eventually, your journey will allow you to be like the lioness that didn't need a menu to follow or a course in Nutrition 101 to eat instinctively. The lioness didn't need to be told that her way of eating was or was not scientifically proven, because her response to and innate desire for meats made her food selections an evidence-based concept. She was an innate instinctive eater—and you will have learned to be an innate instinctive eater also.

Now you are ready to select your blood type options and begin. The next chapter contains your specific eating plan.

## Monitor Your Progress

| Body Signpost | Current Condition | End of Four Weeks | Test Results |
|---|---|---|---|
| 1. Cholesterol level | / | / | |
| 2. Blood pressure | / | / | |
| 3. Low blood sugar or hypoglycemia (yes/no) | | | |
| 4. Body weight | lbs. | lbs. | Lost ___ lbs. |
| 5. Body fat percentage | % | % | |
| 6. Energy level (high/low) | | | |
| 7. Allergies: Hay fever, sinus, headaches, etc. | | | |
| 8. Digestive symptoms: Gas, bloating, diarrhea, constipation, IBS, GERD, stomach pain, arthritic-like pain, etc. | | | |
| 9. List any medications you are taking for the allergies or digestive symptoms described. | | | |

## RECAP

Simply remember the following:

1. Do your best to follow the four-week test. You deserve to know.

2. Do your best to eat ONLY the beneficial and neutral (if necessary) foods.

3. Do your best to avoid the avoid foods. Remember there are plenty of food choices to choose from. You won't be deprived!

4. Enjoy newfound energy, an improved illness profile, and the relief from digestive discomforts. Now you will know what it is to be an instinctive eater for the rest of your life.

# Chapter 7

# INDIVIDUALIZED EATING PLAN FOR TYPE A

A s you realize by now, your blood type can tell a lot about you. It is a great place to begin when you are trying to choose what to eat. There are a lot of diets on the market. However, none are specifically tailored to an individual's needs. Most are very generic. How many times have you had a friend who could eat certain foods and have no ill effects, but when you ate the same foods, you experienced bloating, weight gain, and other discomforts? We are not all alike. Knowing your blood type and the associated beneficial foods is one further step in being able to personalize a plan of eating.

The following food lists are intended to provide you with the benefits of prior research that indicates which foods tend to be best suited for your blood type. While these lists are not written in stone, they do provide the foundation for a blueprint of foods best suited for each blood type. However, because all individuals vary to some degree in body chemistry, your reaction to each food may vary. Only trial and error will tell you which foods are best for you.

It is important to take notice of adverse reactions to specific foods. Listen to your body. If what you are eating does not agree with you, *stop*. Your body has an instinctive mechanism and knows what its needs are and what it can tolerate. Remove any foods that you are having difficulty digesting immediately. There is no need to force your body to accept food that it instinctively rejects.

These food lists also do not account for the consumption of protein, fat, and carbohydrates as they relate to the body's secretion of glucagon and insulin. For that reason, the menus provided will help you with the balance to insure an anabolic state.

As you review the food lists, keep in mind that the beneficial foods tend to metabolize faster and easier because of blood enzymes. Conversely, avoid foods that do not digest or metabolize well and thus disrupt normal metabolism. It is for this reason I suggest that when you start this regimen you eat as many foods from the beneficial foods as possible, slowly adding neutral foods as you gravitate to your specific goal.

Also, since you may be eating more protein than you are used to, you need to drink plenty of water. Water is the universal solvent that aids in digestion and waste removal. As a rule of thumb, divide your body weight by two, then convert the pounds into ounces of water. This will give you the amount of water you should be drinking each day. Example: 150 pounds ÷ 2 = 75 ounces of water a day.

## The 80/20 Approach

A few hard-core disciplined individuals may be able to handle a night-and-day dietary change. But the majority of people will find chipping away at the mountain of dietary change a better option to go by. This group of people may make six steps forward but two steps backward every so often. They will reach the goal, but it won't be a perfect journey. So before you decide to make a

180-degree turn, trying to make all your dietary changes at one time, you might want to consider my 80/20 approach. It will allow you to enjoy the journey more.

Making dietary changes can be very difficult. All of us have made emotional associations with our food choices. We may have established an elaborate reward-and-punishment system: *If I'm good for three days, I can reward myself with that.* Or, *If I cheat once, I can't have that for a whole month or more.* Or you may be an emotional eater—not necessarily eating out of hunger but more as a coping skill for handling your emotions.

Physiological factors like sugar addiction may make it difficult for you. This is common and due to a constant over-response of insulin, which robs the blood of its sugar, causing low blood sugar and promoting a craving for sweets. Generally, sugar addiction occurs from eating too many carbohydrates, particularly an overabundance of simple sugars that are not compatible to your blood type.

Sometimes making dietary changes is difficult simply because of poor eating habits—like late-night eating, skipping breakfast, or eating fast foods.

Whatever the reasons, there is a greater likelihood that you will be successful if you work your way up the path methodically. Keep working until you can successfully choose and eat foods compatible to your blood type 80 percent of the time. Choose the remaining 20 percent of your food selections for taste. Of course, I would prefer that all of us could make proper food choices 100 percent of the time, but we cannot do that—so relax.

Give yourself the benefit of the doubt. Don't place undue stress on yourself and potentially risk your long-term success. That is why I am suggesting my 80/20 approach to instinctive eating. It allows for a gradual adjustment and will feel more realistic. In this way you will make instinctive eating more adaptable to your permanent lifestyle. If you will follow this plan, before long you will find that the 20 percent has shrunk to 15 percent or less.

## PUTTING IT INTO ACTION

Throughout this book I've covered all the "technical" information. Now it's time for you to put all this information to work. It's simple. Just follow the steps below.

### Meal planner

Make copies of the Meal-Planner Chart in Appendix B. The structure of your food plan is outlined below:

- Breakfast

- Snack

- Lunch

- Afternoon snack

- Dinner

- Evening snack

- Before bedtime—Body Genetics Protein Shake (See Appendix A.)

This may seem like a lot of food. However, eating good, healthy food at several sittings during the day helps to keep your metabolism revving at its maximum. Conversely, if you ate six times a day, consuming sugary, high-carbohydrate foods, you would no doubt gain weight and feel extremely sluggish.

## Beneficial and neutral lists

Highlight all the foods you like or are familiar with from the beneficial and neutral lists. Seeing so many foods highlighted should give you the confidence that you can do this!

## Fill in planner

Fill in your Meal-Planner Chart with the meals that appeal to you in the meal plan section that follows the food lists in this chapter. You can mix and match the meals; they are not listed in any particular order. Any breakfast meal idea can peacefully coexist with any lunch or dinner from the list. Or you can create your own meals.

Since I am blood type O, I will show you an example of what my day's selection might look like. All meals are picked from the meal outline section for type Os.

| | Sample Daily Plan #1 | | |
|---|---|---|---|
| **DAY** | **Breakfast** | **Lunch** | **Dinner** |
| 1 | #9<br>Tex-Mex Omelet | #5<br>Grilled beef cheeseburger | #12<br>Roasted pheasant |
| | **Snack #1** Apple and almond butter | **Snack #5** Rice cake | **Snack #11** Almond Bomb Smoothie |

Some meals are picked from the meal outline section, and others are my own creation. You are not confined to the meals that I have suggested.

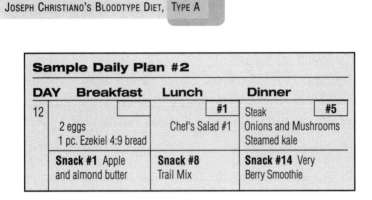

**Sample Daily Plan #2**

| DAY | Breakfast | Lunch | Dinner |
|---|---|---|---|
| 12 | | **#1** | Steak **#5** |
| | 2 eggs | Chef's Salad #1 | Onions and Mushrooms |
| | 1 pc. Ezekiel 4:9 bread | | Steamed kale |
| | **Snack #1** Apple and almond butter | **Snack #8** Trail Mix | **Snack #14** Very Berry Smoothie |

Now, you're ready to begin. Here are the beneficial foods, neutral foods, and foods to avoid for people with blood type A, followed by fourteen days' worth of meal ideas for breakfast, lunch, dinner, and snacking.[1]

# Blood Type A
## Grocery List of Beneficial Foods

### Meats—all anabolic
- [ ] None

### Seafood—all anabolic
- [ ] Carp
- [ ] Cod
- [ ] Grouper
- [ ] Mackerel
- [ ] Monkfish
- [ ] Ocean salmon
- [ ] Pickerel
- [ ] Rainbow trout
- [ ] Snapper
- [ ] Sardines
- [ ] Sea trout
- [ ] Silver perch
- [ ] Snail
- [ ] Tilapia
- [ ] Whitefish
- [ ] Yellow perch

### Beans/legumes
- [ ] Adzuki
- [ ] Black
- [ ] Black-eyed peas
- [ ] Green
- [ ] Lentils, domestic, green, red
- [ ] Pinto
- [ ] Soy, black, brown, green edamame*

### Eggs/dairy
- [ ] Soy cheese*
- [ ] Soy milk
- [ ] Body Genetics Protein Shake*

### Nuts/seeds
- [ ] Flaxseeds
- [ ] Organic peanut butter
- [ ] Pumpkin seeds
- [ ] Redskin peanuts, unsalted

### Oils
- [ ] Linseed (flaxseed)
- [ ] Olive

### Cereals
- [ ] Amaranth
- [ ] Kasha

### Breads
- [ ] Millet bread
- [ ] Ezekiel 4:9 bread
- [ ] Flour, rice, oat, rye
- [ ] Rice cakes
- [ ] Sprouted wheat

### Pastas/grains
- [ ] Artichoke pasta
- [ ] Kasha
- [ ] Oat flour
- [ ] Rice flour
- [ ] Rice pasta
- [ ] Soba noodles
- [ ] Spelt noodles

### Vegetables
- [ ] Alfalfa sprouts
- [ ] Artichokes
- [ ] Beet leaves
- [ ] Broccoli
- [ ] Broccoli sprouts
- [ ] Carrots
- [ ] Chicory
- [ ] Collard greens
- [ ] Dandelion greens
- [ ] Escarole
- [ ] Garlic
- [ ] Horseradish
- [ ] Kohlrabi
- [ ] Leek
- [ ] Okra
- [ ] Onions, red, Spanish, yellow

- Parsley
- Parsnips
- Pumpkin
- Romaine lettuce
- Spinach
- Swiss chard
- Tempeh*
- Tofu*
- Turnips

## Fruit

- Apricot
- Blackberries
- Blueberries
- Boysenberries
- Cherries
- Cranberries
- Figs, dried, fresh
- Grapefruit
- Lemons
- Pineapple
- Plums, dark green, red
- Prunes
- Raisins

## Juice

- Apricot
- Black cherry
- Carrot
- Celery
- Grapefruit
- Pineapple
- Prune

## Spices/condiments

- Barley malt
- Blackstrap molasses
- Garlic
- Ginger
- Miso
- Mustard
- Shoyu
- Soy sauce
- Tamari

## Beverages

- Coffee, regular, decaf
- Green tea
- Red wine
- Water, alkaline
- Water with lemon

## Herbal teas

- Alfalfa
- Aloe
- Burdock
- Chamomile
- Echinacea
- Fenugreek
- Ginger
- Ginseng
- Hawthorn
- Milk thistle
- Rose hips
- Saint John's wort
- Slippery elm
- Strawberry leaf
- Valerian

* Anabolic (higher in protein than
  carbohydrates)

# BLOOD TYPE A
## GROCERY LIST OF NEUTRAL FOODS

### Meats—all anabolic
- ❑ Chicken
- ❑ Cornish hens
- ❑ Turkey

### Seafood—all anabolic
- ❑ Abalone
- ❑ Mahimahi
- ❑ Ocean perch
- ❑ Pike
- ❑ Porgy
- ❑ Sailfish
- ❑ Sea bass
- ❑ Shark
- ❑ Smelt
- ❑ Sturgeon
- ❑ Swordfish
- ❑ Tuna, albacore
- ❑ Weakfish
- ❑ White perch
- ❑ Yellowtail

### Beans/legumes
- ❑ Broad
- ❑ Cannellini
- ❑ Jicama
- ❑ Peas, green pod, snow
- ❑ Snap
- ❑ String
- ❑ White

### Eggs/dairy
- ❑ Eggs*
- ❑ Farmer's cheese*
- ❑ Feta cheese*
- ❑ Frozen yogurt, low fat
- ❑ Goat cheese*
- ❑ Mozzarella, low fat*
- ❑ Ricotta, low fat*
- ❑ String cheese*

- ❑ Goat milk
- ❑ Kefir
- ❑ Yogurt, low fat

### Nuts/seeds
- ❑ Almond butter*
- ❑ Chestnuts
- ❑ Filberts*
- ❑ Hickory*
- ❑ Lychee
- ❑ Pecans
- ❑ Poppy seeds
- ❑ Sesame seeds
- ❑ Sunflower butter
- ❑ Sunflower seeds
- ❑ Tahini (sesame butter)
- ❑ Walnuts*

### Oils
- ❑ Canola
- ❑ Cod liver

### Cereals
- ❑ Barley
- ❑ Buckwheat
- ❑ Cornflakes
- ❑ Cream of Rice
- ❑ Kamut
- ❑ Oat bran
- ❑ Oatmeal
- ❑ Puffed millet
- ❑ Puffed rice
- ❑ Rice bran
- ❑ Spelt

### Breads
- ❑ Brown rice
- ❑ Corn muffins
- ❑ Finn Crisp crispbread
- ❑ Gluten-free bread
- ❑ Oat-bran muffins

- ☐ Oatmeal
- ☐ Rye bread, 100 percent
- ☐ Rye Crisps
- ☐ Ryvita crispbread and crackers
- ☐ Spelt bread
- ☐ Wheat bagels

**Pastas/grains**

- ☐ Cornmeal
- ☐ Flour, barley, bulgur, wheat, graham, spelt, sprouted wheat
- ☐ Quinoa
- ☐ Rice, basmati, brown, white, wild
- ☐ Spelt pasta

**Vegetables**

- ☐ Arugula
- ☐ Asparagus
- ☐ Avocado, Florida
- ☐ Bamboo shoots
- ☐ Beets
- ☐ Bok choy
- ☐ Brussels sprouts
- ☐ Caraway
- ☐ Cauliflower
- ☐ Celery
- ☐ Chervil
- ☐ Coriander (cilantro)
- ☐ Corn, white, yellow
- ☐ Cucumber
- ☐ Daikon
- ☐ Endive
- ☐ Fennel
- ☐ Ferns
- ☐ Green olives
- ☐ Green onions
- ☐ Kale
- ☐ Lettuce, Bibb, iceberg, mesclun
- ☐ Mushrooms, abalone, enoki, portobello, tree oyster, shiitake
- ☐ Mustard greens
- ☐ Radicchio
- ☐ Radishes
- ☐ Rappini
- ☐ Rutabaga
- ☐ Scallion
- ☐ Seaweed
- ☐ Shallots
- ☐ Sprouts, mung, radish
- ☐ Squash, all types
- ☐ Water chestnuts
- ☐ Watercress
- ☐ Zucchini

**Fruits**

- ☐ Apples
- ☐ Black currants
- ☐ Dates
- ☐ Elderberries
- ☐ Gooseberries
- ☐ Grapes, black, concord, green, red
- ☐ Guava
- ☐ Kiwifruit
- ☐ Kumquat
- ☐ Limes
- ☐ Loganberries
- ☐ Melon, casaba, canang, Christmas, crenshaw, musk, Spanish
- ☐ Nectarines
- ☐ Peaches
- ☐ Pears
- ☐ Persimmons
- ☐ Pomegranates
- ☐ Prickly pears
- ☐ Raspberries
- ☐ Star fruit
- ☐ Strawberries
- ☐ Watermelon

**Juices**

- ☐ Apple
- ☐ Apple cider
- ☐ Cranberry
- ☐ Cucumber
- ☐ Grape
- ☐ Vegetable

# BLOOD TYPE A
## GROCERY LIST OF NEUTRAL FOODS (CON'T.)

### Beverages
- ❑ White wine

### Herbal teas
- ❑ Chickweed
- ❑ Colts foot
- ❑ Dandelion
- ❑ Dong quai
- ❑ Elder
- ❑ Gentian
- ❑ Goldenseal
- ❑ Hops
- ❑ Horehound
- ❑ Licorice root
- ❑ Linden
- ❑ Mulberry
- ❑ Mullein
- ❑ Parsley
- ❑ Peppermint
- ❑ Raspberry
- ❑ Raspberry leaf
- ❑ Sage
- ❑ Sarsaparilla
- ❑ Senna
- ❑ Shepherd's purse
- ❑ Skullcap
- ❑ Spearmint
- ❑ Strawberry leaf
- ❑ Thyme
- ❑ Vervain
- ❑ White birch
- ❑ White oak bark
- ❑ Yarrow

### Spices/condiments
- ❑ Agar
- ❑ Almond extract
- ❑ Anise
- ❑ Arrowroot
- ❑ Basil

- ❑ Bay leaf
- ❑ Bergamot
- ❑ Brown rice syrup
- ❑ Brown sugar
- ❑ Cardamom
- ❑ Carob
- ❑ Chervil
- ❑ Chives
- ❑ Chocolate
- ❑ Cinnamon
- ❑ Clove
- ❑ Coriander (cilantro)
- ❑ Corn syrup
- ❑ Cornstarch
- ❑ Cream of tartar
- ❑ Cumin
- ❑ Curry
- ❑ Dill
- ❑ Dulse
- ❑ Honey
- ❑ Horseradish
- ❑ Jam/jelly, from appropriate fruit
- ❑ Kelp
- ❑ Maple syrup, pure
- ❑ Mint
- ❑ Mustard, dry
- ❑ Nutmeg
- ❑ Oregano
- ❑ Paprika
- ❑ Parsley
- ❑ Peppermint
- ❑ Pimiento
- ❑ Rice syrup
- ❑ Rosemary
- ❑ Saffron
- ❑ Sage
- ❑ Salt
- ❑ Savory
- ❑ Spearmint

85

- ❏ Stevia**
- ❏ Sucanat**
- ❏ Tamarind
- ❏ Tapioca
- ❏ Tarragon
- ❏ Thyme
- ❏ Turmeric
- ❏ Vanilla
- ❏ White sugar

\* Anabolic (higher in protein than
  carbohydrate)
\*\* Natural herbal sweetener

# BLOOD TYPE A
## LIST OF FOODS TO AVOID

### Meats

- Beef
- Buffalo
- Duck
- Goose
- Heart
- Lamb
- Liver
- Mutton
- Partridge
- Pheasant
- Pork, all
- Rabbit
- Veal
- Venison
- Quail

### Seafood

- Anchovy
- Barracuda
- Beluga
- Bluefish
- Bluegill bass, sea
- Catfish
- Caviar
- Clams
- Conch
- Crab
- Crayfish
- Eel
- Flounder
- Frog
- Gray sole
- Haddock
- Hake
- Halibut
- Herring, fresh, pickled
- Lobster
- Lox (smoked salmon)
- Mussels
- Octopus
- Oysters
- Scallop
- Shad
- Shrimp
- Sole
- Squid (calamari)
- Striped bass
- Tilefish
- Turtle

### Beans/legumes

- Copper
- Garbanzo (chickpeas)
- Kidney
- Lima
- Navy
- Red
- Tamarind

### Eggs/dairy

- American cheese
- Blue cheese
- Brie
- Buttermilk
- Camembert
- Casein
- Cheddar
- Colby
- Cottage cheese
- Cream cheese
- Edam
- Emmenthal
- Gouda
- Gruyere
- Ice cream
- Jarlsberg
- Milk, skim, 2 percent, whole
- Monterey Jack
- Muenster
- Neufchâtel
- Parmesan
- Provolone

87

- Sherbet
- Sour cream, nonfat
- Swiss cheese
- Whey

### Nuts/seeds

- Brazil
- Cashews
- Pistachio

### Oils

- Corn
- Cottonseed
- Peanut
- Safflower
- Sesame

### Vegetables

- Cabbage, red, white, Chinese
- Eggplant
- Mushrooms, domestic
- Olives, black, Greek
- Peppers, red, yellow, green, jalapeno
- Potatoes, red, white, sweet
- Tomatoes
- Yams

### Fruit

- Bananas
- Coconuts
- Mangoes
- Melons, cantaloupe, honeydew
- Oranges
- Papaya
- Plantains
- Rhubarb
- Tangerines

### Cereals

- Cream of Wheat
- Familia
- Farina
- Granola
- Grape-Nuts
- Wheat germ

- Shredded wheat
- Wheat bran

### Breads

- Seven grain
- English muffins
- High-protein bread
- Pumpernickel
- Wheat-bran muffins
- Wheat matzos
- Whole-wheat bread

### Pastas/grains

- Semolina pasta
- Spinach pasta
- White flour
- Whole-wheat flour

### Spices/condiments

- Capers
- Gelatin
- Ketchup
- Mayonnaise
- Pepper, black, peppercorn, white, red pepper flakes
- Pickles, all kinds
- Relish, all kinds
- Tabasco sauce
- Vinegar, apple cider, balsamic, red, white, red pepper flakes
- Wintergreen
- Worcestershire sauce

### Juice

- Orange
- Papaya
- Tomato

### Beverages

- Beer
- Liquor
- Seltzer water
- Sodas

### Herbal teas

- Black tea, regular, decaf

# BLOOD TYPE A 14-DAY
## PICK-A-MEAL BREAKFAST OPTIONS

### Hot cereal*    1

- 4 oz. vegetable juice
- Medium bowl of oatmeal with soy milk
- ¼ chopped apple and raisins
- 4–5 chopped walnuts
- 1 piece brown rice bread with whole-fruit jam
- 10–12 oz. coffee or strawberry leaf tea

### Hot cereal*    2

- 3 oz. black cherry juice
- Medium bowl of oatmeal made with soy milk
- Blackberries, blueberries, or raspberries
- 4–5 chopped filberts
- 1 piece Ezekiel 4:9 bread with whole-fruit jam
- 10–12 oz. coffee or strawberry leaf tea

### Hot cereal*    3

- 3 oz. prune juice
- Medium bowl of kasha (hot) with soy milk
- 4–5 walnuts
- ½ chopped pear
- 1 piece sprouted wheat bread with almond butter
- 10–12 oz. coffee or green tea

### Pancakes*    4

- 2 medium spelt and walnut pancakes
- Blueberries, blackberries, or strawberries
- Pure maple syrup
- Side of ricotta cheese
- 10–12 oz. coffee or green tea

### Dry cereal*    5

- 4 oz. pineapple chunks
- Medium bowl of spelt flakes with soy milk
- 1 piece 100 percent rye bread with almond butter
- 10–12 oz. coffee or strawberry leaf tea

### Nut butter*    6

- ½ grapefruit or 4 oz. grapefruit juice
- 1 Ezekiel 4:9 bagel
- Organic peanut butter and whole-fruit jam
- 10–12 oz. coffee or green tea

### Smoothie*    7

- Almond Bomb Smoothie (page 101)
- 1 piece Ezekiel 4:9 or millet bread with whole-fruit jam
- 2 plums
- 10–12 oz. green tea or peppermint tea

### Smoothie*     8

- Vanilla Cherry Smoothie (page 103)
- 1 piece 100 percent rye or millet bread with whole-fruit jam
- 10–12 oz. coffee or green tea

### Eggs*     9

- ½ grapefruit
- 2 poached eggs
- Steamed asparagus
- 1 piece rye toast with whole-fruit jam
- 10–12 oz. coffee or green tea

### Eggs*     10

- 4 oz. vegetable juice
- *Cheese Omelet*
    2 scrambled eggs with scallions
    Soy cheese or goat cheese
- Corn muffin with whole-fruit jam
- 10–12 oz. coffee or green tea

### Eggs*     11

- *Salmon Scrambled Eggs*
    2 scrambled eggs
    Crumpled salmon pieces
- Alfalfa sprouts
- 2 sliced kiwifruit
- 1 piece Ezekiel 4:9 or millet bread with whole-fruit jam
- 10–12 oz. green tea or chamomile tea

### Tofu*     12

- *Spanish-Style Scrambled Tofu*
    2 squares firm tofu
    Chopped onion
    Pinch of cumin and oregano
- 1 slice soy cheese
- 1 piece 100 percent rye bread with whole-fruit jam
- 10–12 oz. coffee or green tea

### Cheese*     13

- 4 oz. apricot juice or 20–30 grapes
- Raw carrots, celery, zucchini
- 4 oz. farmer's or feta cheese
- Rye Crisps or Ryvitas
- 10–12 oz. coffee or rose hip tea

### Cheese     14

- 1 apple or pear
- *Grilled Cheese*
    2 pieces sprouted wheat bread
    4 oz. farmer's cheese
- 10–12 oz. peppermint tea or green tea

---

\* Anabolic (higher in protein than carbohydrates)

# Blood Type A 14-Day
## Pick-a-Meal Lunch Options

### Tofu*     1

- *Stir-Fry Tofu*

    1 square tofu

    Broccoli, carrots, zucchini, asparagus, and bamboo shoots
- Shoyu, tamari, or soy sauce
- 10–12 oz. iced peppermint tea or green tea

### Tofu*     2

- Miso soup
- 1 square grilled tofu
- Asparagus and carrots
- Side of brown rice
- 10–12 oz. ginger or green tea

### Tempeh*     3

- *Tempeh Open-Face Sandwich*

    Grilled or baked tempeh

    1 slice soy cheese

    Mushrooms and onions

    1 piece Ezekiel 4:9 bread
- 10–12 oz. green tea or iced ginger tea

### Tempeh*     4

- *Tempeh in Cheeseless Basil Pesto*

    Grilled tempeh

    1 cup cooked spelt or artichoke pasta

    Cheeseless Basil Pesto (page 120)
- Small side salad
- 10–12 oz. iced peppermint tea or ginger tea

### Chicken*     5

- 6–8 oz. roasted chicken
- Roasted parsnips and pumpkin
- Mixed greens with pimiento, cucumbers, and scallions
- Herb Mock Vinaigrette Dressing (page 123)
- 10–12 oz. soda water or green tea

### Seafood*     6

- 6–8 oz. snapper in lemon and dill
- Spinach or collard greens
- Side of parsnips
- 10–12 oz. green tea or Tazo Refresh Tea (peppermint, spearmint, and tarragon blend)

### Seafood*     7

- Miso soup
- 6 oz. canned tuna or sockeye salmon
- Raw spinach and arugula
- Pumpkin seeds and alfalfa sprouts
- Creamy Avocado Dressing (page 121)
- 10–12 oz. iced green tea or ginger tea

### Seafood*     8

- Grilled grouper with lemon
- Watercress, fennel salad with sliced peaches or nectarines
- Raspberry Mock Vinaigrette Dressing (page 124)
- 10–12 oz. green tea or iced raspberry leaf tea

91

## Beans 9

- Lentil dal
- Side of basmati rice
- Blanched asparagus
- 10–12 oz. green tea or iced peppermint tea

## Soup and sandwich 10

- Italian Minestrone Soup (page 106)
- *Tuna Sandwich*

  6 oz. albacore tuna, celery, minced onions (use Creamy Garlic Dressing [page 122] as a mayonnaise substitute)

  2 pieces Ezekiel 4:9 bread
- Lettuce
- 10–12 oz. green tea or spearmint tea

## Mixed* 11

- *Chef's Salad*

  1 hard-boiled egg

  2 oz. turkey or chicken

  2 oz. soy cheese

  ¼ cup soybeans

  Raw spinach and arugula
- Creamy Garlic Dressing (page 122)
- 10–12 oz. green tea or iced peppermint tea

## Turkey* 12

- *Turkey Meatball Parmigiana*

  2 turkey "meatballs" (100 percent turkey meat)

  1 slice mozzarella or soy cheese
- Raw spinach and arugula
- Cucumbers and alfalfa sprouts
- Herb Mock Vinaigrette Dressing (page 123)
- 10–12 oz. bottled water or green tea

## Turkey* 13

- *Mock Waldorf Salad*

  4 oz. sliced turkey

  4–5 chopped walnuts

  ½ chopped apple or pear
- Mesclun salad
- Herb Mock Vinaigrette Dressing (page 123)
- 10–12 oz. green tea or iced peppermint tea

## Turkey* 14

- *Thanksgiving Salad*

  6 oz. cubed turkey

  Appropriate lettuce and dandelion greens, red onion, cucumber, and alfalfa sprouts
- Warm Cranberry Dressing (page 126)
- 10–12 oz. alkaline water or green tea

* Anabolic (higher in protein than carbohydrates)

# BLOOD TYPE A 14-DAY
## PICK-A-MEAL DINNER OPTIONS

### Tofu*      1

- Herbed Tofu (page 110)
- 2 oz. appropriate cheese
- Redskin peanuts or macadamia nuts
- Ryvitas or Rye Crisps
- Small side salad with Miso Dressing (page 124)
- 10–12 oz. ginger tea or iced peppermint tea

### Tempeh*      2

- Grilled marinated tempeh
- Sautéed collard greens, Swiss chard, and kale
- Side of brown rice or quinoa
- 10–12 oz. ginger tea or peppermint tea

### Cheese*      3

- 1 cup butternut, acorn, or other appropriate squash
- 3–4 oz. Mozzarella cheese
- Steamed broccoli
- 3–4 oz. turkey chunks
- Small side salad with appropriate dressing
- 10–12 oz. green tea or seltzer water

### Seafood*      4

- Fish With Herbs and Lime (page 116)
- Side of broccoli and cauliflower
- Side of millet
- 10–12 oz. green tea or alkaline water

### Seafood*      5

- 8 oz. grilled grouper with lemon
- Steamed asparagus and carrots
- Side of quinoa
- 10–12 oz. green tea or alkaline water

### Seafood*      6

- 6–8 oz. grilled marinated fresh tuna steak
- 1–2 artichokes, steamed
- Small side salad with soybeans
- Miso Dressing (page 124)
- 10–12 oz. green tea or glass of red wine

### Seafood*      7

- Broiled salmon with lemon, white wine, and tarragon
- Steamed broccoli
- Side of beets
- 10–12 oz. green tea or glass of white wine

### Turkey*      8

- Turkey burger
- 1 slice appropriate cheese
- Sliced Spanish onion and avocado
- Small side salad
- Creamy Garlic Dressing (page 122)
- 10–12 oz. alkaline water or iced peppermint tea

93

### Turkey*    9

- Roasted turkey
- Roasted carrots, parsnips, onions, and beets with rosemary
- Side of cranberries
- Chestnuts or pumpkin seeds
- 10–12 oz. green tea or alkaline water

### Cornish hen*    10

- 6–8 oz. roasted or grilled Cornish hen
- Side of wild rice
- Small side salad with beets, broccoli, and fennel
- Red Onion Dressing (page 125)
- 10–12 oz. alkaline water or iced peppermint tea

### Chicken*    11

- 4–6 oz. stir-fry chicken
- Stir-fry appropriate vegetables
- Side of edamame
- Side of brown rice
- 10–12 oz. green tea or bottled water

### Chicken*    12

- 6–8 oz. broiled chicken in lemon and white wine
- Brown rice and wild rice (half-and-half blend suggested)
- Steamed broccoli
- 10–12 oz. green tea or bottled water

### Chicken*    13

- Lemon-ginger glazed chicken
- Basmati rice with almond slivers and currants
- Side of brussels sprouts
- 10–12 oz. green tea or ginger tea

### Beans    14

- *Sautéed Swiss Chard and Cannellini Beans*

    Swiss chard sautéed in vegetable stock and onions

    ¾ cup cannellini beans
- 1 cup cooked artichoke pasta
- 10–12 oz. green tea or spearmint tea

* Anabolic (higher in protein than carbohydrates)

# Blood Type A 14-Day
## Pick-a-Meal Snack Options

**Fruit**     **1**

- Large apple with almond butter
- 10–12 oz. green tea

**Fruit\***     **2**

- 1 apple
- 4–6 whole walnuts
- 10–12 oz. green tea or peppermint tea

**Grains/nuts**     **3**

- Unsalted redskin peanuts
- 10–12 oz. ginger tea

**Grains/nuts\***     **4**

- 4–6 walnuts
- 4–5 figs, dried or fresh
- 10–12 oz. green tea or peppermint tea

**Grains/nuts\***     **5**

- Oat-bran muffin
- 1 peach
- 10–12 oz. green tea or chamomile tea

**Trail mix**     **6**

- Apple "Pie" Trail Mix (page 127)
- 10–12 oz. green tea or peppermint tea

**Trail mix**     **7**

- Peanut Chocolate Trail Mix (page 127)
- 10–12 oz. green tea or spearmint tea

**Dairy\***     **8**

- 6 oz. low-fat yogurt
- 1 peach
- 10–12 oz. green tea or ginger tea

**Dairy\***     **9**

- Fresh strawberries with low-fat yogurt
- 10–12 oz. green tea or chamomile tea

**Dairy\***     **10**

- Fresh blueberries and raspberries with low-fat yogurt
- 10–12 oz. green tea or chamomile tea

**Smoothie\***     **11**

- Almond Bomb Smoothie (page 101)

  or

- Apricot Cream Smoothie (page 102)

**Smoothie\***     **12**

- Chocolate Raspberry Smoothie (page 102)

**Smoothie\***     **13**

- Vanilla Cherry Smoothie (page 103)

**Smoothie\***     **14**

- Cranberry Crush Smoothie (page 102)

\* Anabolic (higher in protein than carbohydrates)

## Blood type A—foods that stimulate weight loss

- Vegetable oils—prevent water retention and aid digestion

- Soy foods—metabolize rapidly and aid digestion

- Vegetables—aid digestion and increase intestinal mobility

- Pineapple—increases calorie utilization and intestinal mobility

## Blood type A—foods that cause weight gain

- Meat—stores as fat, increases digestive toxins, and digests poorly

- Dairy foods—inhibit nutrient metabolism

- Kidney beans, lima beans—slow metabolic rate and interfere with digestive enzymes

- Wheat—overabundance impairs calorie utilization

Note: Inhibited insulin production causes hypoglycemia, a lowering of blood sugar after meals, and leads to less efficient metabolism of foods.

# Chapter 8

# PICK-A-MEAL RECIPES FOR TYPE A

THE MOST IMPORTANT thing to remember when following any food plan is to make the food you eat interesting and delicious. If you are not enjoying what you put in your mouth, it really doesn't matter how healthy the food is. You won't eat it again. I know I wouldn't! That is why I have dedicated this next chapter to give you delicious recipes specific to your type A blood. You might actually find a variation of your favorite dish in there modified to suit your blood type. I promise you that you will not have to eat dull, bland, or boring foods in order to implement this program in your life.

If you are a member of a family with varying blood types, I'd like to refer you back to the main book, *Bloodtype, Bodytypes, and You*, where I have included careful cross-referencing in the master index of the recipe section to insure those families with mixed blood types can peacefully coexist. Also in *Bloodtypes, Bodytypes, and You*, you will see that each recipe is marked with the blood types that it was meant for.

Eating healthily does not have to be boring. In fact, on your journey to good health you will no doubt find many new and interesting foods that you otherwise would never have experienced. The key to healthy eating is really to be a bit daring and try new things.

## Master Recipe Listing for Blood Type A

- Almond Bomb Smoothie
- Almond Honey Cookies
- Apple "Pie" Trail Mix
- Apple Crisp
- Applesauce Raisin Muffins
- Apricot Cream Smoothie
- Basic Trail Mix #1
- Basmati Rice Pudding
- Broiled Portobello Mushrooms
- Carob Almond Cookies
- Carrot Bisque
- Cheeseless Basil Pesto
- Cherry Clafouti
- Chicken and Artichokes in Wine Sauce
- Chicken in Garlic Sauce
- Chocolate Mousse
- Chocolate Raspberry Smoothie
- Chocolate Ricotta Cream
- Collard Greens With Nuts
- Corn-Crusted Fish
- Cranberry Crush Smoothie
- Creamy Avocado Dressing
- Creamy Cilantro Lime Dressing
- Creamy Garlic Dressing
- Creamy Squash Bisque

- Dandelion Greens and Leek Frittata
- Earthy Muesli
- Fish With Herbs and Lime
- French Herb Crust
- Greek Herb Crust
- Green Goddess Dressing
- Herb Mock Vinaigrette Dressing
- Herbed Tofu
- Honey Chicken With Lime
- Italian Herb Crust
- Italian Minestrone
- Jerusalem Artichoke Soup
- Lemon-Lime Cilantro Dressing
- Licorice Smoothie
- Maple Magic Smoothie
- Marinated Tuna Steaks
- Middle Eastern Dressing
- Miso Dressing #1
- Miso Dressing #2
- Moroccan Spice Rub
- Onion Soup
- Oregano Feta Dressing
- Peaches and Cream Smoothie
- Peanut Butter Cookies
- Peanut Chocolate Trail Mix
- Pizza Sauce

- Poached Peaches
- Purple Passion Smoothie
- Raspberry Mock Vinaigrette Dressing
- Red Onion Dressing
- Rosemary Chicken
- Sesame Chicken
- Sesame Turkey Fillets
- Soy Cheese Sauce
- Spinach and Mushroom Frittata
- Spinach Pesto
- Sunflower Pancakes
- Tofu Almondine
- Tofu Burgers
- Tofu in Cilantro Sauce
- Tofu Steak Teriyaki
- Traditional Herb Crust
- Turkish Red Lentil Soup
- Vanilla Cherry Smoothie
- Very Berry Smoothie
- Viennese Coffee Smoothie
- Vinegarless Dressing
- Warm Cranberry Dressing
- White Bean and Escarole Soup
- Yummy Rice Pudding

## PICK-A-MEAL RECIPES FOR TYPE A BLOOD*

### MUFFINS

### Applesauce Raisin Muffins

2 cups spelt flour
1 Tbsp. baking powder
1 tsp. cinnamon
½ tsp. nutmeg
¼ tsp. cloves
1 egg

1 egg white
2 cup vanilla soy milk
2 Tbsp. canola oil
⅓ cup honey
¾ cup unsweetened applesauce
½ cup raisins or black currants

Preheat oven to 400 degrees. Line muffin tin with paper liners.

In large bowl, mix together flour, baking powder, cinnamon, nutmeg, and cloves. Mix well. In another bowl, beat egg and egg white. Add soy milk, canola oil, honey, applesauce, and raisins. Mix well.

Fold wet mixture into flour mixture. Mix until combined. Spoon batter into tins, and bake for 20–25 minutes. *Makes 12 muffins.*

---

### PANCAKES

### Sunflower Pancakes

1 cup oat flour
½ cup spelt flour
2½ tsp. baking powder
1 egg

1 tsp. honey
1 cup soy milk
2 Tbsp. apricot juice
¼ cup sunflower seeds

Combine flour and baking powder in large bowl. Mix well. In another bowl lightly beat egg. Add honey, milk, and apricot juice to egg. Fold wet mixture into dry mixture. Add sunflower seeds. Mix until combined.

Ladle ¼ cup batter onto nonstick griddle. Cook until surface begins to bubble. Flip and allow other side to cook for another 2 minutes. *Makes 12 pancakes; 1 serving = 3 pancakes.*

---

* Unless otherwise noted in Notes section, all recipes are courtesy of Joseph Christiano, author.

## CEREAL

### Earthy Muesli

2 cups rolled oats
1 cup rye flakes
1 cup coarsely chopped dates
1 cup raisins or black currants
1 cup coarsely chopped filberts
½ cup coarsely chopped walnuts

½ cup sunflower seeds
½ tsp. nutmeg
1 tsp. cinnamon
1 tsp. vanilla or almond extract
4 cups apple cider

Combine all dry ingredients in large bowl. Mix well. Place mixture in airtight storage container. Slowly stir in vanilla or almond extract and apple cider.

Place in refrigerator overnight with container sealed tightly. Ready to eat in morning! *Makes 4–5 servings; 1 serving = 1 average cereal bowl.*

## SMOOTHIES

For all the recipes below, place ingredients into blender and process until smooth. If they come out too thick for your liking, just add more designated liquid or some water.

### Almond Bomb

1 cup soy milk
4 ice cubes
1 tsp. almond extract
1 tsp. almonds, crushed or
  slivers, as garnish

1 scoop vanilla Body Genetics
  Protein Shake *(blood type
  specific)*

## Apricot Cream

1 cup soy milk
3–4 frozen or canned apricot
halves
2–3 ice cubes
2 cup silken soft tofu

1 tsp. vanilla extract
1 scoop vanilla Body Genetics
Protein Shake *(blood type
specific)*

---

## Chocolate Raspberry

1 cup soy milk
½–¾ cup frozen raspberries
½ cup silken soft tofu

1 scoop chocolate Body
Genetics Protein Shake
*(blood type specific)*

---

## Cranberry Crush

½ cup frozen blueberries
½ cup frozen cranberries
½ cup soft silken tofu
1 tsp. vanilla extract

1 tsp. honey
½ cup cranberry juice
1 scoop Body Genetics Protein
Shake *(blood type specific)*

---

## Licorice

1 cup soy milk
2–3 ice cubes
¼ tsp. licorice root (can be
adjusted for taste)
½ cup vanilla low-fat yogurt or
2 cups silken soft tofu

1 scoop vanilla Body Genetics
Protein Shake *(blood type
specific)*

---

## Maple Magic

1 cup soy milk
3–4 ice cubes
2 tsp. pure maple syrup
½ cup vanilla low-fat yogurt or
    silken soft tofu

1 scoop vanilla Body Genetics
    Protein Shake (*blood type
    specific*)

## Peaches and Cream

1 cup soy milk
½ cup vanilla low-fat yogurt
1 sliced frozen peach

2–3 ice cubes
1 scoop Body Genetics Protein
    Shake (*blood type specific*)

## Purple Passion

1 cup concord grape juice
½ cup vanilla low-fat yogurt or
    silken soft tofu

3–4 ice cubes
1 scoop Body Genetics Protein
    Shake (*blood type specific*)

## Vanilla Cherry

1 cup soy milk
½ cup vanilla low-fat yogurt or
    silken soft tofu
2–3 ice cubes

½ cup frozen cherries
1 scoop Body Genetics Protein
    Shake (*blood type specific*)

## Very Berry

1 cup soy milk
½–¾ cup frozen berries
    (raspberries, blueberries,
    strawberries)

2–3 ice cubes
1 scoop vanilla Body Genetics
    Protein Shake (*blood type
    specific*)

## Viennese Coffee

1 cup soy milk
2–3 tsp. instant coffee
½ tsp. cinnamon or nutmeg
3–4 ice cubes

1 scoop vanilla Body Genetics Protein Shake *(blood type specific)*

---

## SOUPS

### Carrot Bisque

1 lb. sliced carrots
1 large chopped onion
¾ cup chopped parsnips
2 minced shallots
1–2 cloves minced garlic

2 bay leaves
2 Tbsp. olive oil
2 Tbsp. mellow white miso
2–3 tsp. fresh chopped parsley or dill to garnish

In large saucepan, sauté carrots, onion, parsnips, shallots, garlic, and bay leaves in olive oil for 3–4 minutes. Add water to cover vegetables. Water level should be 1½ inches above vegetables. Bring to boil. Reduce to simmer and cook until vegetables are soft.

Ladle 1 cup liquid into bowl. Dissolve miso in this liquid. Add more hot liquid if necessary. Once incorporated, add miso mixture back to soup pot. Stir well. (Miso should never be boiled. It is added at end of preparation of dish and replaces salt in soup.)

Remove from heat. Purée with hand blender to desired consistency. Stir in parsley or dill. Soup can be strained through sieve if you prefer creamier soup. *Makes 4–6 servings.*

---

## Creamy Squash Bisque

2–3 lbs. winter squash (butternut, acorn, delicata), skin removed and cubed
1 small diced onion
1 tsp. fresh finely minced ginger
1 diced carrot
1 stalk diced celery
2 Tbsp. olive oil
5 cups vegetable stock
½ cup apple juice
½ tsp. nutmeg
Parsley for garnish

Preheat oven to 450 degrees. Cut squash in half. Lay squash cut side down on cookie sheet. Bake for 35–45 minutes. Check doneness with a fork. Set aside to cool for few minutes.

In large saucepan, sauté onions, ginger, carrot, and celery in olive oil for 5–7 minutes, or until onions are translucent. Add stock, apple juice, and nutmeg. Scoop out pulp from squash and add to the mix. Stir well.

Let cook for 10 minutes more. Use hand blender to purée soup into creamy bisque. Toss parsley into soup, and serve immediately. *Makes 6–8 servings.*

## Italian Minestrone

1 medium diced onion
1–2 cloves minced garlic
2 diced carrots
½ cup winter squash cut in ¼-inch cubes (acorn, butternut, etc.)
2 stalks diced celery
2 Tbsp. olive oil
1 cup fresh packed spinach, kale, or escarole

1 16-oz. can cannelloni beans (or other appropriate bean)
¼ cup chopped fresh parsley
6 cups chicken stock
½ cup spelt pasta elbows or other small pasta shape
½ cup diced zucchini
1 cup sliced green beans
3–4 sliced basil leaves

In large saucepan, sauté onion, garlic, carrots, squash, and celery in olive oil for 3–4 minutes. Add spinach (escarole or kale), beans, parsley, and stock. Simmer for 10–15 minutes. Meanwhile, cook pasta al dente. Rinse well and set aside.

Add zucchini, green beans, and cooked pasta. Cook until all vegetables are soft. Stir basil into finished soup. Let cook for 1 minute more. Serve. *Makes 6–8 servings.*

## Jerusalem Artichoke Soup

1 lb. Jerusalem artichokes
Lemon juice from half a lemon
4 Tbsp. butter or olive oil
2 sliced leeks, white part only

2 sliced carrots
3 cups chicken stock
Pinch of salt
1 lb. silken tofu

Scrub Jerusalem artichokes well. (If they are scrubbed well you will not need to peel them.) Slice them, and blend with lemon juice in bowl.

In medium saucepan, melt butter. Add leeks, carrots, and artichokes. Cover and cook over low heat for 20–25 minutes. Add 2½ cups chicken stock and pinch of salt. Cover and cook for 30 minutes more.

Purée remaining stock with silken tofu. Add to pot until combined. Soup can be strained through sieve if you prefer smoother soup. *Makes 4 servings.*

## Onion Soup

1 Tbsp. butter or olive oil
2 red onions
2 white onions
2 yellow onions
2 leeks
3 shallots
Small head of peeled garlic
3 cans chicken stock

1 bay leaf
1 tsp. thyme
1 tsp. savory
¾ cup red wine
Optional: appropriate bread with slice of appropriate cheese

Melt butter or oil in large soup pot. Sauté onions, leeks, shallots, and garlic on low heat for about 30 minutes. Add stock, seasonings, and wine. Let cook for another 45 to 60 minutes. Put cheese on bread. Place in bottom of each individual bowl. Pour hot soup into bowl and serve. *Makes 6 servings.*

## Turkish Red Lentil Soup

2½ cups dry red lentils
1 large minced onion
2 cloves minced garlic
2 diced carrots
1 diced celery stalk
2 Tbsp. olive oil

4–6 cups vegetable stock
½ tsp. salt
Juice from 2 lemons
1 cup chopped fresh spinach or Swiss chard, stems and ribs removed

Place lentils in bowl. Cover with cool water. Let stand in water until softened.

In large saucepan, sauté onion, garlic, carrots, and celery in olive oil for 3–4 minutes. Rinse lentils and remove from water. Add to saucepan. Add vegetable stock and salt. Liquid level should be 2 inches above ingredients. Use more water if needed. Bring to boil, then lower to simmer. Let cook for 25–35 minutes, or until lentils are cooked. Remove from heat.

Slowly add half the lemon juice to pot. Let sit for 5 minutes. Taste. Add more lemon juice as desired. For a really lemon taste, add entire amount. Mix in spinach or chard. Heat of soup will wilt greens. *Makes 6–8 servings.*

## White Bean and Escarole (or Swiss Chard) Soup

2 Tbsp. olive oil
1 small diced onion
2–3 cloves smashed garlic
1 16-oz. can cannellini beans
(or other appropriate white bean)
4–5 cups water

2 Tbsp. mellow white miso
2 Tbsp. rosemary, fresh or dried
Salt to taste
½ lb. escarole or Swiss chard, trimmed and coarsely chopped

Heat olive oil in large soup pot. Sauté onion and garlic for 3–5 minutes. Add beans and cook until warm.

Heat 1 cup water. Dilute miso in warm water. Set aside.

Purée ⅔ of onions and beans in food processor. Slowly add miso water to thin beans. The consistency should be somewhat loose. Add more water if necessary.

Add puréed beans to soup pot with whole beans and onion. Add balance of water, rosemary, and salt to taste. Bring to simmer. (Note: Miso should never be boiled. It breaks down easily under high temperatures.) Add escarole or Swiss chard. Cook for 10 minutes more. Serve immediately. *Makes 4–6 servings.*

## EGGS

### Dandelion Greens and Leek Frittata

1½ lb. dandelion greens
5–6 cups water
3–4 Tbsp. olive oil
2 cloves finely minced garlic
1 cup chopped leeks, white part
  only

6 eggs
2 Tbsp. fresh chopped parsley,
  or 1 Tbsp. dry parsley
Pinch of salt
4 artichoke hearts, sliced

Wash dandelion greens. In large pot, bring water to boil. Put dandelion greens into pot to cook for 3–4 minutes. Remove from pot. Pat away excess water. Coarsely chop. (This will remove some bitterness. If you don't mind bitter taste, skip the parboil stage.)

Using half the oil, sauté garlic and leeks in large nonstick skillet until leeks start to soften. Add dandelion greens to skillet. Cover and let cook for about 10 minutes. Remove from heat. Drain any excess liquid from skillet. Set aside.

Beat eggs, parsley, and salt in large bowl. Add dandelion mixture to egg mixture, along with artichoke hearts. Mix well.

Reheat skillet over medium heat with remaining oil. Be sure oil is hot before adding eggs and greens to skillet. Cover and let cook for 5–8 minutes or until bottom browns. DO NOT turn eggs during cooking process. When cooked, place large plate or platter over top of skillet. Turn over to flip frittata onto plate. Serve warm or cold. *Makes 3–4 servings.*

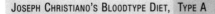
## Spinach and Mushroom Frittata

3–4 Tbsp. olive oil
2–3 cloves finely minced garlic
1 cup chopped leeks, white part only
4 cups chopped mushrooms (*blood type specific*)

1 lb. spinach
6 eggs
2 Tbsp. fresh chopped parsley, or 1 Tbsp. dry parsley
½ tsp. nutmeg
Pinch of salt

Using half the oil, sauté garlic and leeks in large nonstick skillet until leeks start to soften. Add mushrooms and sauté for 3 minutes. Add spinach to skillet. Cover and let cook for about 10 minutes. Remove from heat. Drain excess liquid from skillet. Set aside.

In large bowl, whisk eggs until fluffy. Add parsley, nutmeg, and salt. Add spinach mixture to egg mixture. Mix well. Reheat skillet over medium heat with remaining oil. Be sure oil is hot before adding eggs and greens to skillet. Cover and let cook for 5–8 minutes or until bottom browns. DO NOT turn eggs during cooking process.

When cooked, place large plate or platter over top of skillet. Turn over to flip frittata onto plate. Serve warm or cold. *Makes 3–4 servings.*

## TOFU

## Herbed Tofu

1 lb. firm tofu
1 tsp. plum paste (umeboshi paste)
1 tsp. lemon juice
2 tsp. tahini

1–2 tsp. each of 4 or 5 of the following dried herbs: oregano, basil (use fresh if possible), parsley (use fresh if possible), dill, marjoram, tarragon

Drain tofu. Crumble and set aside. In large bowl, cream plum (umeboshi) paste, lemon juice, and tahini together. Add tofu and stir well. Fold in herbs. Chill and serve. *Makes 4–5 servings.*

## Tofu Almondine

⅓ cup soy sherry
⅓ cup soy sauce
⅓ cup fresh lemon juice
3 fresh packed oregano leaves
1 lb. firm or extra-firm tofu
2 cups cooked white rice

4 cups water
1½ cups chopped portobello
   mushrooms
⅓ cup toasted, coarsely
   chopped almonds

Combine sherry, soy sauce, lemon juice, and oregano leaves. Set aside ¼ cup of marinade for cooking mushrooms separately. Drain tofu. Place between several layers of paper-towel thicknesses to absorb extra liquid. Begin to cook rice with water. Place tofu in nonstick skillet over medium-low heat. Add all marinade, except for ¼ cup set aside. Cook tofu until heated through. In another nonstick skillet, add ¼ cup marinade and mushrooms. Simmer for 10 minutes or until mushrooms are cooked. Serve tofu on top of rice. Garnish with almonds. *Makes 4 servings.*

---

## Tofu Burgers

1 lb. extra-firm tofu, drained
   well
½ cup cooked brown rice
½ cup dry breadcrumbs
½ cup chopped scallions
2 egg whites

¼ cup grated carrots
½ cup low-fat mozzarella or soy
   cheese
2 tsp. soy sauce
2 tsp. ground walnuts (optional)

Mash tofu. Mix all ingredients thoroughly. Form burgers. Heat nonstick skillet to medium with spray of olive oil. Cook burgers until golden. *Makes 6 servings.*

---

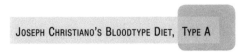
## Tofu in Cilantro Sauce

If you have never tried tofu, this is the recipe to start with. Even non-tofu eaters love it! Serve over steamed greens with appropriate grain. It's even good cold as part of a salad.

1 lb. firm or extra-firm tofu
2 Tbsp. canola or olive oil
1 tsp. fresh finely minced ginger
2 cloves finely minced garlic
½–¾ cup fresh cilantro, packed and finely chopped

1–2 Tbsp. soy, tamari or shoyu sauce
2–3 Tbsp. water
1–2 Tbsp. honey

Drain tofu well. Let it sit on plate with another plate on top of it. Weigh top plate down with large can of vegetables from your cupboard while you are preparing all other ingredients. This will help excess water to leave tofu. However, be careful not to smash tofu block. Cut tofu into 4 equal squares.

In large nonstick skillet, heat oil on medium heat. Add ginger and garlic. Sauté for 1 minute. Do not burn. Add tofu. Be sure to place tofu directly on ginger and garlic. Let cook for 2–3 minutes. Turn tofu squares over.

Add cilantro, soy sauce, and 2 tablespoons water. Drizzle honey over entire mixture. Cover and let cook for 2–3 minutes. Stir well. Add more water if sauce is too thick. Remove from skillet and serve. *Makes 4 servings.*

---

## Tofu Steak Teriyaki

1 lb. extra-firm tofu, drained well
6 Tbsp. sake or white wine
2 medium cloves crushed garlic
6 Tbsp. soy sauce

4 Tbsp. olive oil
2 chopped scallions
2 Tbsp. honey
1 Tbsp. arrowroot

Slice tofu into six equal ½-inch strips. Marinate tofu in sake or wine, garlic, soy sauce, 2 tablespoons olive oil, scallions, and honey. Heat remaining oil in wok over medium heat. Grill tofu in wok until brown on both sides. Bring leftover marinade to boil. Lower to simmer for 2 minutes. Thicken sauce with arrowroot. *Makes 4–5 servings.*

---

## CHICKEN

### Chicken and Artichokes in Wine Sauce

4 boneless chicken breasts, skinned and cut in half
¼ cup spelt flour or other appropriate flour
4 Tbsp. olive oil
1 tsp. dried thyme
1½ tsp. dried rosemary
Pinch of oregano
2–3 cloves finely minced garlic
½ cup white wine
½ cup chicken broth
3–4 sliced artichoke hearts, packed in water
¼ cup fresh parsley, chopped

Rinse chicken and pat dry. Dredge chicken in flour. Heat 2 tablespoons olive oil in large nonstick skillet over medium-high heat. Cook chicken 3 minutes on each side.

Reduce heat. Add dried herbs to skillet with remainder of olive oil. Distribute herbs evenly. Add wine, chicken broth, and artichoke hearts to the pan. Cover and let simmer for 10 minutes. Stir in parsley to finish dish. *Makes 4 servings.*

---

### Chicken in Garlic Sauce

1 lb. chicken fillets, cut into bite-size chunks
2 cups broccoli florets
1 cup asparagus
2 Tbsp. olive oil
2–4 cloves minced garlic
2 Tbsp. grated fresh ginger
2 Tbsp. fresh lemon juice
½ cup chopped scallions (optional)
Dash of hot chili oil

Rinse chicken in cold water and pat dry.

Steam broccoli florets and asparagus in large covered pot for 5 minutes. Use 1 inch of water on bottom of pot to create steam.

Heat olive oil in large skillet or wok. Sauté garlic and ginger for 1 minute. Add chicken and lemon juice. Cook for 3–4 minutes. Add broccoli and asparagus to skillet (also add scallions if using). Simmer for 4–5 minutes until chicken and vegetables are cooked through. *Makes 3–4 servings.*

---

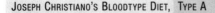
## Honey Chicken With Lime

½ tsp. garlic powder
4 boneless, skinless chicken
   breast halves
⅓ cup pineapple juice
¼ cup honey

1 tsp. lime zest
3 Tbsp. fresh lime juice
2 Tbsp. soy sauce
2 tsp. corn starch

Sprinkle garlic powder over chicken; let sit while you prepare sauce.

In small bowl, whisk together pineapple juice, honey, lime zest, lime juice, and soy sauce until well mixed. Brush chicken with sauce. Heat large nonstick skillet to medium heat. Cook each piece of chicken 5 minutes on each side or until done.

Bring leftover marinade to boil. Lower to simmer for 2 minutes. Thicken sauce with cornstarch. *Makes 4 servings.*

---

## Rosemary Chicken[1]

6 cloves of crushed garlic
2 Tbsp. fresh or dried rosemary
Juice of 4 limes (about ½ cup)
½ cup olive oil

½ tsp. salt
1 quartered chicken (3½–4 lbs.)
4 rosemary sprigs for garnish
1 lime sliced for garnish

In large bowl, combine garlic, rosemary, lime juice, olive oil, and salt. Place quartered chicken in bowl. Turn to coat all pieces. Cover with plastic wrap and marinate in refrigerator for 3 hours. Turn chicken once during marinating time.

Heat cast-iron skillet to hot. Add chicken pieces, and weight them down with heavy lid or another cast-iron skillet. Cook until crispy, 15 minutes on each side. Serve chicken, garnished with sprig of rosemary and wedge of lime. *Makes 4 servings.*

---

## Sesame Chicken

1 lb. chicken, cut up
2 Tbsp. tamari, shoyu or light
   soy sauce
2 Tbsp. water

1 tsp. honey
½ Tbsp. fresh minced ginger
2 Tbsp. canola oil
1 Tbsp. toasted sesame seeds

Rinse chicken in cold water. Pat dry.

In small bowl, combine tamari sauce, water, honey, and ginger. Whisk together and set aside.

Heat canola oil in large skillet. Cook chicken 1 minute on each side. Add tamari mixture to chicken. Let cook until mixture comes to slight boil and thickens somewhat. Remove chicken from skillet. Sprinkle with toasted sesame seeds. *Makes 2 servings.*

---

## TURKEY

## Sesame Turkey Fillets

1 lb. turkey fillets
2 Tbsp. tamari, shoyu or light
   soy sauce
2 Tbsp. water

1 tsp. honey
½ Tbsp. fresh minced ginger
2 Tbsp. canola oil
1 Tbsp. toasted sesame seeds

Rinse turkey fillets in cold water. Pat dry.

In small bowl, combine tamari sauce, water, honey, and ginger. Whisk together and set aside.

Heat canola oil in large skillet. Cook turkey 1 minute on each side. Add tamari mixture to turkey. Let cook until mixture comes to a slight boil and thickens somewhat. Remove turkey from skillet. Sprinkle with toasted sesame seeds. *Makes 2–3 servings.*

---

## FISH/SEAFOOD

### Corn-Crusted Fish

1 cup finely ground cornmeal
1 tsp. dried parsley
1 tsp. dried dill
½ tsp. salt

1½ lb. fresh cod (or any firm,
   white fish)
1 Tbsp. olive oil
Sliced lemons or limes

Combine cornmeal with parsley, dill, and salt. Mix well. Dredge cod in cornmeal mixture.

Heat skillet with olive oil. Add fish to skillet, and cook over medium heat for 5–7 minutes per side. Use cover so that fish will cook through. (Cooking time will depend on thickness of fish. Fish is done when it begins to flake.)

Just before fish is cooked completely, add a few tablespoons of water to skillet. Allow fish to finish cooking with lid on pan. Remove fish from pan, and garnish with sliced lemons or limes. *Makes 3–4 servings.*

---

### Fish With Herbs and Lime[2]

1½ lb. fresh red snapper or cod
¼ cup lime juice (not from
   concentrate)
4 garlic cloves, pressed or
   minced
½ cup chopped fresh parsley

½ cup chopped scallions
1 tsp. chopped fresh rosemary,
   or ½ tsp. dried rosemary
1 tsp. fresh thyme, or ½ tsp.
   dried thyme
1 tsp. sweet paprika

Preheat oven to 375 degrees. Rinse fish in cold water and pat dry. In medium bowl, mix together lime juice, garlic, parsley, scallions, rosemary, thyme, and paprika. Place fish in nonstick baking dish (unoiled) and spread topping evenly over fish. Cover tightly with foil, and bake for 25 minutes until fish flakes with a fork. *Makes 3–4 servings.*

---

## Marinated Tuna Steaks

⅓ cup olive oil
¼ cup tamari, shoyu or light
   soy sauce
Lemon juice from half a lemon
2 cloves smashed garlic

2 Tbsp. fresh chopped coriander (cilantro)
1 dollop honey
4 tuna steaks (6 oz. each)

Combine all ingredients except tuna in large Ziploc bag or in shallow bowl. (Ziploc bag makes it easier to move marinade around the fish.) Mix ingredients well. Add tuna to marinate. Cover tuna completely with mixture. Place in refrigerator for 15–30 minutes. Use this time to prepare other parts of your dinner.

Grill or broil tuna steaks on medium heat to desired doneness, 3–4 minutes per side for rare, 5 minutes for medium-well. Let fish sit for 5 minutes before serving. *Makes 3–4 servings.*

---

## VEGETABLES

## Broiled Portobello Mushrooms

1 Tbsp. balsamic vinegar
2 Tbsp. water
3–4 Tbsp. olive oil
Pinch of salt
1 Tbsp. fresh chopped parsley

1 lb. whole portobello mushrooms, stems removed
1 lb. spinach
1 oz. goat cheese per mushroom

Preheat broiler.

In small bowl, combine vinegar, water, oil, salt, and parsley. Brush cleaned mushrooms with marinade. Place on baking sheet, cap side up. Broil for 3–5 minutes or until mushrooms soften.

Place trimmed and cleaned spinach in large saucepan of boiling water. Let boil for 3 minutes. Leaves should just turn bright green. Do not overcook. Remove from water and set aside.

Turn mushrooms over, apply more marinade, and place some crumbled goat cheese inside cap. Let broil until cheese starts to bubble and brown. Remove. Serve mushrooms on bed of spinach. *Makes 4 servings.*

---

## Collard Greens With Nuts

1 cup raisins
1 cup boiling water
¼ cup crushed walnuts or
    almond slivers

2 cloves finely minced garlic
1–2 Tbsp. olive oil
1 lb. collard greens

Soak raisins in boiling water for 10 minutes. In small skillet, toast nuts over medium heat for 4–5 minutes. No oil is necessary. In large saucepan sauté garlic in oil over low heat until soft, about 2–3 minutes. Raise heat to medium. Add collards to garlic. Sauté for 4–5 minutes. Add reserved raisin-soaking water. Cover and let steam for 10–15 minutes or until collards are tender. Stir in raisins and serve. *Makes 4 servings.*

## SPICE RUBS AND HERB CRUSTS

One of the easiest ways to increase the flavor of tofu, meat, fish, and poultry is to use dry spice rubs or herb crusts. Any of these mixtures can be used dry, or add 1 teaspoon of water to create a paste. Fresh herbs are suggested unless otherwise specified.[3]

## Morroccan Spice Rub

1 Tbsp. chopped fresh mint
2 cloves minced garlic
2 tsp. grated fresh ginger

½ tsp. ground cinnamon
½ tsp. ground red pepper

*Makes about 3½ tablespoons.*

## French Herb Crust

3 Tbsp. chopped fresh parsley
1 Tbsp. chopped fresh chives
2 tsp. chopped fresh thyme

2 cloves minced garlic
2 tsp. grated lemon rind

*Makes about 5 tablespoons.*

### Greek Herb Crust

2 Tbsp. chopped fresh parsley
1 Tbsp. chopped fresh oregano

1 Tbsp. grated lemon rind
2 cloves minced garlic

*Makes about 4 tablespoons.*

### Italian Herb Crust

3 Tbsp. chopped fresh parsley
2 Tbsp. chopped fresh basil

2 cloves minced garlic
2 tsp. grated lemon rind

*Makes about 5 tablespoons.*

### Traditional Herb Crust

2 Tbsp. chopped fresh parsley
1½ Tbsp. chopped fresh
    rosemary

2 cloves minced garlic

*Makes about 3½ tablespoons.*

## SAUCES

### Cheeseless Basil Pesto

6–8 whole almonds
2–3 cloves garlic
1 Tbsp. light miso
5–6 cups fresh basil leaves,
  packed, trimmed, and
  stemmed

⅓ cup extra-virgin olive oil
Pinch of salt
1 Tbsp. fresh lemon juice

In food processor, pulverize almonds and garlic. Add in miso and pulse lightly. Slowly add basil leaves one cup at a time to processor with a little oil. Continue this process until all oil and basil are incorporated.

Taste pesto and adjust seasoning if necessary with pinch of salt. If you like looser pesto, add more olive oil. However, a paste consistency is OK too. It's up to your personal preference.

Add lemon juice to preserve color of basil. Extra pesto can be frozen in small container. *Makes about ¾–1 cup.*

### Pizza Sauce

2 tsp. sugar
1 tsp. salt
2 tsp. paprika
1 tsp. oregano powder
1 tsp. dried basil
1 tsp. dried parsley

1 tsp. dried thyme
2 tsp. onion powder
1 tsp. garlic powder
3 drops anise flavoring
½ cup water

In small bowl, combine all dry ingredients and mix well. Stir in anise flavoring and water. Mix well. *Makes about ½ –1 cup.*

## Soy Cheese Sauce

3 oz. cheddar soy cheese
3 oz. silken tofu
1 Tbsp. soy milk or water

2 Tbsp. vegetable oil (linseed,
canola, or olive)

Grate soy cheese, and combine everything in microwave-safe bowl. Heat on high for 30 seconds, then blend well with hand blender. Repeat this step until cheese is melted and mixture is completely combined. *Makes 1–1½ cups.*

---

## Spinach Pesto

1 bag fresh spinach (350 grams),
stemmed and trimmed
½ cup packed fresh basil leaves
or a sprinkling of dried basil
1 Tbsp. extra-virgin olive oil

4 cloves pressed garlic
1 Tbsp. pine nuts *(optional)*
½ tsp. sea salt
1–2 oz. feta cheese

In large stainless-steel pot, heat ½ inch of water. Toss in spinach and cover. Let steam for 1–2 minutes. Spinach should just be wilted, not completely cooked. Remove from pot and drain immediately.

Place spinach and all other ingredients in food processor. Purée thoroughly. Pesto can be stored in container in freezer or refrigerator. *Makes about 1–1½ cups.*

---

## Creamy Avocado Dressing

4 oz. soft silken tofu
½ ripe avocado *(blood type
appropriate)*
Juice of 1 lemon

1 tsp. soy sauce
¼ cup water
Salt to taste

Place all ingredients in food processor. Purée until smooth. Add water, 1 tablespoon at a time, to thin as necessary. *Makes 1½ cups.*

---

## Creamy Cilantro Lime Dressing

1 cup plain low-fat yogurt
1½ Tbsp. fresh chopped cilantro
1½ Tbsp. finely minced scallions or chives

1 Tbsp. fresh lime juice
1 tsp. honey (optional)
Pinch of salt

In small bowl or food processor, combine all ingredients until smooth. Add water as needed, 1 teaspoon at a time. Let sit in refrigerator for at least 1 hour so flavors can blend. *Makes 1 cup.*

## Creamy Garlic Dressing

1½ cups plain low-fat yogurt
1 Tbsp. almond butter
1 Tbsp. fresh lemon juice

2 cloves minced garlic
1 Tbsp. fresh or dried parsley
Pinch of salt

In small bowl or food processor, combine all ingredients until smooth. Add water as needed, 1 teaspoon at a time. *Makes 1½ cups.*

## Green Goddess Dressing

4 oz. silken tofu
2 Tbsp. Braggs Liquid Amino
1 tsp. brown rice syrup or honey

¼ cup fresh chopped parsley
2–4 fresh chopped basil leaves
1 Tbsp. fresh chopped chives

Bring small saucepan of water to boil. Add tofu; simmer for 5 minutes. Drain well. Set aside to cool for several minutes. Place cooked tofu and all other ingredients in food processor. Purée until smooth. Add water, a teaspoon at a time, to thin if necessary. *Makes 1–1½ cups.*

## Herb Mock Vinaigrette Dressing

½ cup fresh lemon juice (about 3–4 lemons)
¼ cup Braggs Liquid Amino
1 cup cold-pressed olive oil
1 cup cold-pressed canola oil (or other blood type appropriate oil—not flax)

1 clove pressed garlic
1 tsp. dried mustard
1 tsp. dried basil, or 1 Tbsp. fresh basil
1 tsp. dried tarragon
½ tsp. dried parsley, or 1 tsp. fresh parsley

Combine all ingredients in jar or plastic container with lid. Seal tightly and shake vigorously to blend. *Makes 1 cup.*

---

## Lemon-Lime Cilantro Dressing

1 dollop honey
Juice of 1 lemon
Juice of ½ lime
¼ cup tamari, shoyu, or light soy sauce

¾ cup olive oil
2 cloves smashed garlic
2–3 Tbsp. fresh chopped coriander (cilantro)

Place honey in small bowl. Set bowl in larger bowl of hot water. Heat will loosen honey up. Once it is loose, add citrus juices, tamari, and olive oil. Whisk together well. Add garlic and coriander. Whisk well. Let sit at room temperature for 1 hour so flavors can blend. *Makes 1 cup.*

---

## Middle Eastern Dressing

1½ cups plain low-fat yogurt
1 Tbsp. almond butter
1 Tbsp. fresh lemon juice

1 clove minced garlic
½ tsp. ground cumin
Pinch of salt

In small bowl or food processor, combine all ingredients until smooth. Add water as needed, 1 teaspoon at a time. *Makes 1½ cups.*

---

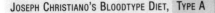
## Miso Dressing #1

½ cup light miso
½ cup olive oil
½ cup water

¼ cup lemon juice
1 tsp. dry mustard

Put all ingredients in food processor and blend well. If you do not have a food processor, bring water to near boil and mix miso until smooth. Whisk in all other ingredients. Let stand at room temperature before serving. *Makes 1¼ cups.*

## Miso Dressing #2

1 Tbsp. sweet white miso
Juice and zest of 1 lemon
2 Tbsp. soy sauce

2 Tbsp. Braggs Liquid Amino
¼ cup olive oil
1 tsp. dried basil

Dilute miso in lemon juice and soy sauce using whisk. Add all other ingredients. Whisk to blend. *Makes 1¼ cups.*

## Oregano-Feta Dressing

2 oz. feta cheese
2 Tbsp. fresh lemon juice
1 Tbsp. olive oil

1 clove crushed garlic
½ tsp. dried crushed oregano

Put all ingredients in food processor and pulse until mixed. *Makes 1 cup.*

## Raspberry Mock Vinaigrette Dressing

6 fresh raspberries
2 Tbsp. Braggs Liquid Amino
1 cup olive oil

1 tsp. finely minced red onions
½ tsp. dried rosemary

Smash raspberries in Braggs Liquid Amino until they are completely broken up. Combine all ingredients in jar or plastic container. Shake vigorously to blend. *Makes 1 cup.*

## Red Onion Dressing

½ cup fresh lemon juice (about
    3–4 lemons)
¼ cup Braggs Liquid Amino
1 cup cold-pressed olive oil
1–2 Tbsp. finely chopped red
    onion

½ tsp. dried mustard
½ tsp. dried oregano or parsley
½ tsp. dried thyme, minced or
    pressed

Combine all ingredients in jar or plastic container. Shake vigorously to blend. Let sit at room temperature for an hour or so before using to allow flavors to blend. *Makes 1½ cups.*

## Vinegarless Dressing

½ cup fresh lemon juice (about
    3–4 lemons)
¼ cup Braggs Liquid Amino
1 tsp. garlic powder
1 cup cold-pressed olive oil

1 cup cold-pressed canola oil
    (or other blood-type appro-
    priate oil—not flax)
1 tsp. minced onions
½ tsp. curry or turmeric

Place all ingredients in quart-sized plastic container with lid and pouring feature. Mix ingredients well. If consistency is too thick, add water, or next time use less olive oil and increase other oil. (Add other spices you would like based on your blood type.) Keep refrigerated for 3–4 weeks. *Makes 2¾ cups.*

## Warm Cranberry Dressing

1½ cup fresh, cleaned cranberries

Lemon juice and zest from 1 lemon

2 Tbsp. brown rice syrup or maple syrup

¼ cup olive oil

1 tsp. fresh finely minced ginger

2 Tbsp. soy sauce

½ tsp. plum paste (umeboshi paste)

¼ cup crushed walnuts for garnish

In food processor, combine cranberries, lemon juice, zest, and syrup. Mix to a minced consistency. If you like it chunkier, adjust to your preference.

Combine oil, ginger, soy sauce, and plum paste in small saucepan over low heat. Once warm, add cranberry mixture. Let simmer for 5–7 minutes. Remove from heat. Serve and garnish with crushed walnuts. *Makes 1½ cups.*

---

## TRAIL MIXES

Trail mixes are an easy, convenient snack. Make a batch to keep in your cupboard. There are many combinations that can be made from your grocery lists. Below we are providing some sample ideas for trail mixes and a simple guideline for creating your own personalized blend. Remember, your trail mix must use ingredients that are blood-type appropriate.

## SUGGESTED TRAIL MIX RECIPE GUIDELINES

Use the measurements given for each component.

| | |
|---|---|
| ½ cup dried fruit | raisins, apples, black currants (Avoid other dried fruits, which are extremely high in sugar.) |
| 1½ cup nuts (anabolic) | walnuts, almonds, hickory, unsalted redskin peanuts, filberts |
| ¼ cup nonanabolic nuts or seeds | pumpkin seeds, sesame seeds, sunflower seeds |
| ½ cup something chocolate | carob chips, chocolate chips |

### Apple "Pie" Trail Mix

¼ cup black currants
½ cup almonds
¼ cup dried apple pieces

¼ cup pumpkin seeds
1 cup walnuts

### Basic Trail Mix #1

½ cup raisins
¼ cup sunflower seeds
¾ cup almond slivers

½ cup carob or chocolate chips
1 cup walnuts

### Peanut Chocolate Trail Mix

¼ cup black currants
½ cup filberts
1 cup unsalted redskin peanuts

½ cup carob or chocolate chip
2 cup almonds

## DESSERTS

### Almond Honey Cookies

1 cup mild, light olive oil
1 2-inch strip lemon peel
½ cup dry white wine
¼ cup honey
1½–2 tsp. grated lemon zest
½ cup sliced almonds or walnuts

1 tsp. almond extract or vanilla
  extract
3½ cups spelt flour *(or other
  appropriate flour)*
1 tsp. cinnamon

In saucepan, gently heat olive oil and lemon peel. Oil should be warm, but not hot enough to "fry" rind. You only need to have oil on heat long enough to warm it. Remove from heat, and place in large mixing bowl to cool. Remove and discard rind once oil has cooled. Add wine, honey, lemon zest, almonds, and extract. Stir gently to mix.

In another bowl, sift together flour and cinnamon. Slowly pour oil mixture into flour mixture, stirring as you go. Once ingredients are incorporated, knead dough with your hands. Let dough rest for 30 minutes in refrigerator.

Preheat oven to 350 degrees. Roll dough into small balls, and flatten with back of a spoon. Bake for 15–20 minutes or until lightly browned. *Makes 12–16 cookies.*

## Apple Crisp

*Filling:*
8 medium apples, sliced
½ cup raisins
¼ cup spelt flour
½ tsp. cinnamon
½ cup apple cider

*Topping:*
1 cup rolled oats
2 Tbsp. spelt flour
⅓ cup light honey
2 Tbsp. canola oil
¾ tsp. cinnamon (optional)
⅓ cup crushed walnuts
  (optional)

Preheat oven to 375 degrees. Spray 2-quart baking dish with cooking spray. In large bowl, place sliced apples and raisins with flour and cinnamon (if using). Toss so apples are coated entirely by flour mixture. Pour into baking dish.

In another bowl, combine all topping ingredients and mix well.

Pour apple cider into baking dish over apples. Crumble topping over apples. Bake for 35–45 minutes or until apples are tender and golden. *Makes 4–6 servings.*

---

## Basmati Rice Pudding[4]

1½ cups uncooked white basmati rice
5 cups water
½ tsp. ground cinnamon
½ tsp. ground cardamom
1¾ cups soy milk

½ tsp. salt
⅓ cup black currants
¼ tsp. pure vanilla extract
⅔ cup honey
¼ cup slivered almonds

Rinse and drain basmati rice. In food processor, chop rice into smaller pieces. Soak overnight in enough water to cover grains.

In large pot, combine 5 cups water, drained rice, butter, cinnamon, and cardamom. Cook on medium heat for about 20 minutes or until rice is soft. Add milk, salt, and black currants. Cook to pudding consistency, stirring frequently. Remove from heat, and let cool for 2–4 minutes. Stir in vanilla, honey, and almonds. Serve immediately. *Makes 4–6 servings.*

---

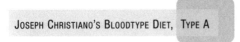
## Carob Almond Cookies

1½ large apples (pears can also be used)
⅓ cup almond butter
2 tsp. canola oil
2 eggs
¼ tsp. unbuffered, corn-free vitamin C crystals
1¼ cups brown rice flour, or 1 cup brown rice flour and ¼ cup spelt or Kamut flour

¾ tsp. baking soda (1 tsp. baking powder can be substituted for vitamin C and baking soda)
¾ cup carob powder
¼ tsp. salt
30 whole almonds (optional)

Preheat oven to 350 degrees. Spray two cookie sheets with cooking spray. Chop apples into small chunks and put in blender. Add almond butter, oil, eggs, and vitamin C. Purée everything together. You may need to push apples down a few times to get them to purée. If necessary, add a little bit of water.

In separate bowl, combine flour, baking soda (or baking powder), carob powder, salt, and almonds (if using). Mix well. Add purée to dry mixture and stir until mixed. Form round teaspoon-size balls and drop onto cookie sheet. Bake for 10–12 minutes. Cookies are done when toothpick inserted comes out slightly moist. Allow to cool for 5 minutes. Refrigerate extras in airtight container. *Makes 6 servings.*

## Cherry Clafouti

¼ cup spelt flour (or other appropriate flour)
½ cup light honey (lavender honey works best)
2 eggs, lightly beaten

2 egg yolks
2 cups appropriate milk at room temperature
½ tsp. vanilla extract
2 cups pitted fresh cherries

Preheat oven to 375 degrees.

Place flour in a large bowl, making well for eggs and yokes. Using a whisk, slowly pour in milk and mix well. Whisk to a smooth consistency. Add honey and vanilla extract. Mix well.

In 8-inch deep-dish pie pan sprayed with cooking spray, evenly distribute fresh cherries. Carefully pour batter mixture over the fruit. Cook for 40–45 minutes or until brown and puffy. Let cool for 10 minutes before serving. *Makes 6 servings.*

---

## Chocolate Mousse

1 10-oz. package firm silken tofu, drained
¼ cup light honey
¼ cup fruit syrup

½ tsp. ground cinnamon
1 tsp. instant coffee
2 tsp. cocoa
½ tsp. vanilla

Place all ingredients in food processor and purée until mixed. Place in airtight container, and refrigerate until well chilled. *Makes 3–4 servings.*

---

## Chocolate Ricotta Cream[5]

1 15-oz. container of low-fat
   ricotta cheese
2 Tbsp. sifted unsweetened
   cocoa powder
5 Tbsp. honey

¼ tsp. cinnamon
½ tsp. vanilla extract
1 Tbsp. toasted sliced almonds
   as garnish

Place ricotta in food processor or blender and process for 1 minute. Add all other ingredients. Purée until smooth and creamy. Adjust sweetness and serve. *Makes 6 servings.*

## Peanut Butter Cookies

1 cup canola oil
1 cup organic peanut butter
1 cup sucanat
1 tsp. vanilla extract
2 eggs
2 cups spelt flour
1 tsp. baking soda
2 Tbsp. soy flour
1 cup oat flour (made from
   freshly ground whole oats in
   food processor)

*Optional:*
½–1 cup of the following:
   organic sunspire chocolate
   chips
   chopped peanuts
   carob chips

Preheat oven to 350 degrees.

In a large bowl, cream oil, peanut butter, and sucanat. Add vanilla and eggs. Stir in baking soda and flour. Combine until well mixed. Fold in any optional ingredients.

Drop tablespoon-size balls onto cookie sheet. Bake for 10–12 minutes. *Makes 2 dozen cookies.*

## Poached Peaches

3 Tbsp. honey or sucanat
1 cup apple cider or red wine
1 cup water
2 whole cloves (optional)
3 thin slices of lemon rind

½ tsp. vanilla extract
6 ripe fresh peaches, firm,
    peeled, pitted and cut in half
    (or pears)
¼ cup black currants (optional)

In large saucepan, combine honey, wine or cider, water, cloves, lemon rind, and vanilla. Submerge peaches and currants in liquid. Try to insure liquid covers fruit as much as possible. Bring to boil. Lower to medium heat; cover and simmer for 15–20 minutes, turning fruit frequently, or until the fruit is soft.

Once cooked, remove fruit from liquid. Boil reserved liquid until it reduces by half. Spoon over cooked fruit and serve. *Makes 4 servings.*

---

## Yummy Rice Pudding[6]

2 apples
¼ cup rolled oats
½ cup apple juice
⅓ cup water
½ cup cooked brown rice
¼ tsp. cinnamon
1 Tbsp. brown rice syrup

Dash of allspice
*Optional garnishes:*
    Sprinkling of toasted
      almonds or walnuts
    Sprinkling of black currants

Peel, core, and slice apples.

Lightly roast oats by stirring them in saucepan over medium heat until they smell toasty. Add apples and other ingredients. Bring to boil. Cover and simmer for 20 minutes.

Blend in blender until smooth. Garnish with desired elements.

---

# Chapter 9

# NUTRITIONAL SUPPLEMENTS FOR BLOOD TYPE A

AS FAR BACK as I can remember, I have always taken nutritional supplements. As a young teenager I would save the money I earned from my paper route and snow-shoveling jobs so I could go to the health food store and buy my supplements. I have always viewed purchasing nutritional supplements as an investment in my health. I am walking proof of those health benefits for more than forty-five years, and by the grace of my heavenly Father I have enjoyed a very healthy quality of life—I feel it, it shows, and it will do the same for you.

Supporting your diet with nutritional supplements is vitally important. Just by virtue of genetic engineering or modifying of food sources, pesticides, chemicals, fertilizers, and waste materials being dumped and pumped into our soil, water, and air, nearly all vegetation as we know it today is lacking in the minerals and elements originally required to help sustain humankind. So even with your best efforts of eating well, you are prone to be deficient in minerals and vitamins. It is a fact that if you were to trace back to the root of nearly every ailment and disease, you would find a mineral deficiency.

That's why, as a naturopathic doctor, I believe it is wise and prudent to first use every natural means possible to get the body to return to normal function so it can heal itself. If medications are to be used, they should be taken for emergency situations after exhausting every natural means available.

When you engage in physical work and recreational activities or embark on a regular exercise program, it is important that you add nutritional supplements and protein to your diet due to the extra demands placed on your body. There are specific supplements you can take when you are planning to lose weight or want to enhance performance for sports. Conditions like heart arrhythmia or elevated cholesterol, to mention just a couple, are benefited with other nutritional supplementation. Consider the stress in your life, the negative side effects of medication, and poor eating habits and choices, and you can see why your body is taking a beating. So I strongly recommend that you consider taking daily supplements.

## Fantastic Help . . . With Limitations

Dietary supplements are not formulated to cure illness or disease, but they do provide the environment for assisting your body in the healing process. They can promote cellular health and systemic and organ function, and they can assist in purifying your body through detoxification and removing toxic buildup so your body can heal itself and be restored to normal health as it was designed to do.

However, nutritional supplements have limitations and can't do it all themselves; they need your help. The benefits that come from taking nutritional supplements can be maximized only when working in concert with healthy living habits. I suggest when deciding to make healthier lifestyle changes that you do not view them as a temporary change but as a way of life. Healthy life choices that work in concert with your nutritional supplements are:

- Diet (eating food compatible to your blood type)

- Drinking enough water (alkaline water)

- Regular exercise

- Proper rest and relaxation

- Daily exposure to sunshine and fresh air

- Physical activities

- Serving and forgiving others

- Positive thoughts

It's all about investing in your health.

## You Need a Healthy Brain

One more consideration I would like to point out regarding your health is the fact that nearly 90 percent of all disease and sickness comes from the brain. This involves the electrical frequencies and magnetism in your body that are necessary for building healthy, functional molecular structures. The brain operates like an electrical generator, causing electricity to flow throughout your entire body, including the liver.

It is important to know that the liver is dependent upon the brain's electricity. Not only does the liver receive the patterned frequencies from the brain in order to function, but it also receives the invaluable magnetic draw for the uptake of mineral energy, particularly calcium. In other words, in order to assimilate the minerals it desperately needs to function, your liver (and other organs) depends on the electrical circuits from the brain.

When there is a disruption or short circuit in the electrical flow to the liver from the brain, the liver is deprived of this magnetism, which in turn sets the stage for degenerative changes in the liver. Like a domino effect, the rest of the body's organs and systems become affected from these short circuits, and you have what is known as the onset of degenerative diseases.

### Mental "dis-ease"

I gave you this microscopic overview of body chemistry to point out that disease and illness are directly related to the altering or short-circuiting of the electrical flow from the brain, especially to the liver. "Dis-ease" is due to the lack of "perfect peace." Anytime your mind lacks peace, it becomes prey to anxieties, frustrations, guilt, phobias, depression, and so on. The most powerful causes of interference of electrical flow to the body, particularly the liver, are worry, fear, lust, self-centeredness, hatred, and bitterness.

Negative mental thoughts contribute to the development of degenerative disease.[1] This is scientific proof and even is confirmed in the Bible, recorded thousands of years ago: "For as he thinks in his heart, so is he" (Prov. 23:7, NKJV). This defective thinking, or negative thoughts, becomes the enemy of truth, and such defective thinking has an effect on your body chemistry. If the ability of your mind to comprehend or understand truth about your health is blocked, for example, it will in a sense cancel the benefits of your health program.

From a physical perspective, the first stages of mental impairment begin with calcium deficiency. Combine that with a carbohydrate imbalance interfering with oxygen to the brain, and you have the formula for mental distortions, resulting in your thinking being unclear and filled with anxiety and fear. As you can tell, healthy lifestyle changes include a change of mind or attitude that involve your entire makeup—body, soul, and spirit.

## Nutrition Support Ideas

We all are in need of nutrition support. Make nutritional supplements a part of your lifestyle, and remember the significance of the word *prevention*. As you experience the many positive healthy benefits from dietary supplementation, you will grow in the wisdom as to why I perceive it as a wise investment in your health.

Below I have given you a brief list of nutrition support ideas and strategies that I believe will cover the bases for most people. They are foundational as far as supporting your diet (compatible with your blood type). Of course, if you have a specific health condition or concern, please consult with your health practitioner or go to my Web site (www.bodyredesigning.com) and click on Ask Dr. Joe. Simply send me an e-mail with your concerns, and I will get back to you as soon as I can.

The following list also represents what I personally take as a means of prevention as well as for cleansing, strengthening, and fortifying my bodily functions and systems for promoting homeostasis or balance. As my needs change, I make adjustments in what supplements I take. I believe these are necessary and worthy of your consideration for additional support to your healthy lifestyle, as we discussed.

## Colon health: detoxification

I strongly recommend that you do a colon cleanse as the first step for improving your health. Before you can ever expect an organ, gland, or bodily system to heal and be restored to natural function, you must detoxify your body. As you start making healthy lifestyle changes to avoid or eliminate illness or any health condition, you must first detoxify your colon. I cannot express this fact strongly enough. The healing process cannot take place if your body is toxic.

A dysfunctional colon plays a major role in most degenerative diseases. A dysfunctional colon is related to a slow transit time, which is the time it takes to eliminate food once it has been ingested. This is generally caused by constipation. If you do not have three bowel movements per day, you may be considered clinically constipated. The transit time of a healthy colon is approximately twenty-four to forty-eight hours. When the transit time is slowed down due to constipation (average American adult transit time is ninety-six hours), a buildup of toxins from impacted fecal matter forms. Mucus and fecal matter that get impacted into the porous walls of the colon not only cause digestive pain and discomfort, but they also lead to more serious conditions such as diverticulitis, IBS, diverticulosis, polyps, and, worse, cancer of the colon.

As the toxins remain in the colon, they eventually get picked up by the bloodstream (a condition called leaky colon) and circulate throughout your body, polluting it and breaking down your quality of health. This condition overloads the liver and causes it to weaken. The health of your colon is directly related to the health of your blood.

Constipation develops from a lack of exercise; not drinking enough water; eating refined flour and refined sugar products, fried foods, and deli food; lack of dietary fiber; and taking medications. (This condition can be improved by making proper lifestyle changes.) Constipation also makes your colon a breeding bed for parasitic infestation. Once these parasites work their way into your colon, they do two things: eat what you ate and excrete their feces into your body while building their breeding colonies. These parasites range from single-cell amoebae to four-inch worms, spreading their toxic refuse throughout your body, which eventually weakens and interrupts your health. Parasitic infestation contributes to a litany of health-related problems like liver dysfunction, degenerative diseases, headaches, achy joints, weakness, weak immune system, skin ailments, poor skin tone, bad breath, and many more.

After you have gone through a colon cleansing, it is necessary to take care of your colon on daily basis to maintain regularity. Since preventing constipation is a daily part of keeping a healthy colon, I strongly suggest that you take a fiber supplement every day of your life. Fiber provides the bulk necessary for speeding up the transit time for proper elimination. It helps prevent the buildup of waste and toxicity in your colon while contributing to lowering your bad cholesterol.

Many people experience chronic constipation, a condition that prevents bowel movement for many days or even weeks at a time. Chronic constipation is a very dangerous condition that promotes illnesses, diminishes normal colon function, enhances parasitic infestation, and causes toxicity buildup, which leads to serious poor health conditions (as mentioned above), not to mention the pain and discomfort associated with chronic constipation. If you are suffering with chronic constipation, I recommend an extra-powerful herbal laxative that provides immediate bowel movement to relieve the discomfort and enhance proper colon function and health. (See www.bodyredesigning.com.)

### Digestive enzymes

It is true that chewing food slowly and thoroughly will allow food to be broken down more efficiently by allowing the enzymes to do their work, but as we age, the body secretes fewer enzymes that are necessary for proper digestion of food. This condition is common for those who are forty and older, causing digestive disorders, poor nutrient uptake, and eventual poor health. To compensate for the natural decline in enzyme production, consider a complex digestive enzyme supplement with every meal. Digestive enzymes will give your liver and digestive system a break and will also assist in eliminating the discomforts associated with poor enzymatic action. A digestive enzyme complex will enhance your body's ability to break down the food you ingest and allow proper nutrient uptake and assimilation. (See www.bodyredesigning.com.)

### Multivitamins

A multivitamin is a means to supplement the nutrition I get from food sources. A balance of vitamins, minerals, and herbs serves as a healthy safety net for prevention. Going to the next level of specificity, I take multivitamins that are compatible with my blood type (O). You would need to take one specifically geared to your type A blood. I recommend a daily multivitamin supplement that comes from food extracts and sources that contain vitamins, minerals, antioxidants, and herbs specifically formulated for the nutritional needs of each individual blood type. (See www.bodyredesigning.com.)

## Minerals

*Trace minerals* are the minute but vital amount of certain minerals that your body does not manufacture; therefore, you need to supply your body with them. We have already discussed the reasons you do not necessarily get them from your food. Without trace minerals, your body cannot absorb vitamins.

I find that a concentrated liquid form is best because I can mix it with water, soups, drinks, or swallow it right from a teaspoon. I have had great success in helping people with dissolving bone spurs and avoiding surgery simply by suggesting they take liquid trace minerals for thirty to sixty days. Strong nails and fast nail growth, better hair condition, and more energy are but a few of the many benefits you will experience when adding trace minerals to your nutritional regimen.

Calcium is priceless. Calcium is an organic mineral and is essential for the function of every organ and gland. It is also necessary for balancing the blood and tissue pH in the body. Calcium is the major mineral our body needs in abundance, yet it is the most difficult mineral to absorb. Calcium needs magnesium and vitamin $D_3$ (cholecalciferol) to be assimilated properly in the body. Here's a way to save some money: spend one hour in direct sunlight, and you will get approximately 50,000 mg of vitamin D—so get out in the sun.

I prefer taking coral calcium from Okinawa. Calcium carbonate and calcium citrate are probably the easiest to assimilate, especially for women. A pregnant woman requires five to seven times more calcium than a man. (See www.bodyredesigning .com.)

## Protein

Protein is essential for your body; your body could not function without it. And you probably are not getting enough protein on a daily basis. The American diet is virtually full of refined white flour products and refined sugars—carbohydrates—all empty and unusable calories. Just by adding protein to your diet and reducing carbohydrates, not only will you see an immediate drop in weight, but you will also experience improved mental alertness and ability to think clearly. If you suffer from hypoglycemia and bouts with low blood sugar, you can restore constant energy and avoid "crashing" in the morning and afternoon when you consume enough protein.

High-protein/no-carbohydrate diets work very well for immediate weight loss, but they can cause you to lose control when carbohydrates are reintroduced to the diet. I wouldn't recommend these diets for a long period of time because your health is dependent on carbohydrates as well.

Of course, the majority of protein should come from food sources, but eating protein is not always palatable or convenient. That's why I recommend considering a protein supplement in the form of a bar or shake. They may serve as a meal replacement or an in-between-meals snack.

When it comes to a protein shake, whey protein is very common because it is not expensive. However, since it is a derivative of dairy (cow's milk), you should avoid it. Soy protein makes for a great shake and is beneficial for blood type A. But if you are allergic to soy, don't use it. Rice milk and almond milk are good alternative sources of protein.

I believe you should use a protein shake that is compatible to your blood type so you can get maximum assimilation and usage from it. I prefer using egg white protein powder with water for my shakes. When I travel, I always take my stash with me—protein powder and protein bars. (See www.bodyredesigning .com.)

## Water—living water

There are basically three causes for disease and death: free-radical damage to cells, dehydrated cells, and acidosis. When you consider that the human body is made up of trillions of cells, it stands to reason that the healthier the cell, the healthier the individual. The baseline solution of our cells (fluid inside and outside the cell) determines their health and function. When free radicals (impaired molecules) attach themselves to cells in the body, those cells break down. Depending on how long cellular damage has occurred, the degree of ill health will be determined. And depending on where the weakened cells are located in your body, you will suffer disease of the liver, heart, blood, or other body systems.

If the cells do not get proper hydration (water) with bioavailable minerals, an imbalance in the cell occurs; the body falls out of homeostasis. Ultimately, this condition may lead to a variety of diseases and eventually death. Additionally, when the intracellular and extracellular fluid pH level becomes overly acidic for too long, the body will experience organ dysfunction, such as that of the gallbladder or liver. This condition is referred to as acidosis.

The root problem in this case is likely that the individual's pH is out of balance (too acidic) because of a deficiency in sodium. A deficiency of other organic minerals such as calcium, potassium, or magnesium is very common too. When we maintain the proper level of minerals in the body through proper hydration, the body has the mineral reserves to protect itself if the pH should go out of balance for various reasons temporarily. We replenish our body with minerals via diet and nutritional supplements. If the mineral reserves are low or depleted, the body will go into a survival mode to protect itself by creating a buffer. It will go to the next available source of minerals to balance its pH, like calcium.

For example, if the body requires calcium, where do you think it gets it? You guessed it—the bones. In order to protect itself, the body will leach calcium from the bones if a state of acidosis remains too long; however, this "robbing" process causes a lack of calcium in the bones, resulting in osteoporosis.

Think about the healthy athlete or fitness enthusiast who suddenly experiences a heart attack. It seems uncanny, but it happens, and I see it happening more and more. After the victim is dead, an examination is usually conducted to determine if there was some kind of gene or rare genetic disorder that caused the unexpected heart attack. However, the root cause could be simpler than that. If the body chemistry was in a state of acidosis caused by dehydration, that athlete or fitness enthusiast would have developed the perfect condition for a sudden heart attack. How could this happen?

Perhaps the level of acidity was further elevated by adding a high-protein pre-workout meal or snack and routinely eating a high-protein diet with foods that leave an acid ash on the tissues, along with the effect of everyday stress. With an ever-increasing acid buildup in the body, the health is constantly challenged. Continuing this lifestyle over time, this healthy-looking athletic man or woman is developing a state of acidosis, which may make him or her the perfect candidate for a heart attack. If you don't learn how to neutralize your pH, the end result will always be damaging to your health, and if it remains undetected, it could become life threatening.

There are a couple of things you can do to neutralize and keep your pH in check. In brief, limit an *acid* ash–like diet, which is basically the result of eating mostly meats, fish, eggs, and cereals, with very little fruit and vegetables in your diet. This kind of diet will produce acidification of the urine. To neutralize this acid condition, add more *alkaline* ash–producing foods such as fruit and vegetables.

You can neutralize the acid and balance your pH by drinking ionized or alkaline water, which is one of my daily practices. As imperative as it is for you to hydrate the cells to keep them healthy and properly functioning, it is equally imperative that you know the type of water you drink. For several years, since the infamous craze for drinking bottled water, I have researched what kind of water is in those bottles. I have discovered that nearly all bottled water is acidic, even if it is purified. If you don't believe me, pick out any of the most popular bottled waters at random and compare them to the findings posted on my Web site at www.bodyredesigning.com.

I tested many bottled waters. In fact, I saw the results of nearly all of them, and I was amazed at the claims by doctors and experts who are selling purified water that is acidic. Just think about this for a minute. Since there is a direct link between your blood and tissue pH and cancers and other known diseases, we can conclude that maintaining the proper pH level is crucial.

Since my research of bottled water, I have made a habit of drinking ionized (alkaline) water exclusively. I have a machine that restructures my tap water into alkaline water. It not only filters out all the chemicals and impurities that make our drinking water unhealthy, but it also retains all the natural bioavailable minerals that are in the water: sodium, calcium, magnesium, and potassium. It reduces the molecular size of the water by half, and through electrolysis, an electrical charge helps drive more alkaline water into my cells. The benefits I get from drinking alkaline water are:

- Neutralizing acid buildup from my workouts

- Neutralizing my pH from foods that leave an acid ash on the tissues

- Hydrating my cells with chemical-free water

- Protecting my cells from free-radical damage

The alkaline water is also a natural antioxidant, which counteracts the potential damage to my cells by free radicals. It supplies my body with plenty of bioavailable minerals and assists in balancing my pH. Please drink water. And make sure you drink alkaline water for your health. (See www.bodyredesigning .com.)

## Natural antiaging hormone (HGH)

There is nothing you can do about the clock on the wall as it continues its relentless, perpetual motion. So when it comes to aging, we all share one thing in common—we're all getting older. However, some of us will make choices that will definitely change the effects of time—we can slow down the aging process.

When I refer to the aging process, I am referring to health-related conditions associated with aging, such as increased body fat, loss of muscle tissue, decreased libido and energy, elevated blood pressure, poor sleep quality, and poor appearance (skin tone), just to mention a few. These common conditions associated with aging can be reversed or slowed down by taking human growth hormone (HGH), preferably in a homeopathic oral form. Other nutritional supplements that are available at www.bodyredesigning.com, such as DHEA, melatonin, HGH Support, and Women's Support, play a vital role as we attempt to slow down the aging process, but allow me to concentrate on HGH for now.

Human growth hormone is critical for our development during childhood and plays a key role in the development of bones, muscles, organs, and the body as a whole. HGH dramatically decreases as you develop to maturity. It is produced naturally by your pituitary gland and other immune cells until you reach your midtwenties. But by the age of eighty, it is virtually nonexistent in your body. The natural aging process affects your overall health and quality of life due to the lack of HGH in your body. Add stress to the formula (which reduces HGH production), and you can see why it's all downhill after you hit thirty to thirty-five years of age.

Since I have been taking this antiaging hormone supplement HGH, I can confirm that it helps me stay leaner, has improved my skin tone, and gives me the satisfaction of knowing I am replacing what my body won't produce anymore. Even my mother takes HGH and comments on the improvement she enjoys in sleeping well each night. If you are over thirty years of age, male or female, I recommend HGH as a part of your nutrition support strategy.

What is listed above is not necessarily mandatory for you to take, because everyone is different. Nor is the list exhaustive, but it does provide a wide spectrum for your consideration. Visit my Web site at www.bodyredesigning.com for a complete list of dietary supplements that range from covering the bases to more specific.

There are no magic bullets, potions, or lotions for improving your health. A healthy life will be a result of creating a balance in your body, soul, and spirit. It encompasses the positive things you do (physical activities), what you ingest (nutrition), the positive thoughts you embrace (forgiveness, compassion for others), keeping a positive attitude (walking in victory), and connecting with your Creator (perfect peace of mind).

## Recap

Simply remember the following:

1. Think "prevention" when you consider taking dietary supplementation.

2. Dietary supplementation is not a cure-all and does have limitations, but when you make healthy living your lifestyle, then you will maximize the benefits from your supplements.

3. Your attitude or point of view toward life is a valuable factor for healthy living, both mentally and physically.

4. Eating correctly for your blood type and exercising regularly are the fitness twins necessary for making your life healthier.

# Chapter 10

## TIPS FOR MAKING IT ALL WORK

**A**FTER LEARNING THE basics I have provided for you in the previous chapters, now it is time to apply the principles to your everyday life. Your goal is to improve, not perfect, your lifestyle so it can be as healthy as possible. Because you are the master of your domain, you should do very well when it comes to preparing meals, snacks, and desserts for family members and yourself.

But what about when you decide to go out and dine? Or perhaps you travel a lot on business and must eat at various restaurants. I am sure you want to be on top of that as well. This approach to eating will surprise you that it is not all that difficult to make it work in your daily routines because after all, you are eventually going to be an instinctive eater and will know what works best for you and what doesn't. Then the decision is just deciding whether you want what works best or not.

Check out the tips below, and see how they can benefit you both at home and out in the real world.

## Tips for Making It at Home

1. *Remove avoid foods.* I suggest removing the foods you love that are on the avoid list from the household immediately. Donate them to charity or to a neighbor. They will be thankful for them.

2. *Plan ahead.* Try to fill in a week's worth of meal planning at first. From your meal plans you can create your shopping lists.

3. *Try something new.* Each week try to incorporate one or two new foods into your meal plans. Try a new dish from the recipe section. You might discover that you really enjoy foods that previously you would not have tried.

4. *Cook your own meals.* This will cut down on the frustration of having your food prepared with spices, condiments, or preservatives that may be undesirable for your type A blood. Food you prepare yourself tastes better. Plus, this will keep some money in your pocket.

5. *Use healthy cooking methods.* Choose your preparation methods carefully to avoid excess saturated fats and undesirable ingredients. Desirable cooking methods include boiled, broiled, baked, steamed, sautéed (light on the oil), grilled, or poached. Undesirable cooking methods include fried, pan-seared, or BBQ (too much sauce).

6. *Rotate foods.* If you eat the same food every day, you are bound to get bored. I would suggest giving yourself a three- to five-day rotation of foods. For example, if you eat amaranth flakes for breakfast on Monday, try not to eat these same flakes until Thursday. There are a variety of other cereals or menu possibilities for you to choose from in the interim. Your taste buds will be happy, and so will your metabolism. If you eat the same foods over and over, your metabolism is not challenged; therefore, it slows down. By giving your body many different varieties of fuel (food), it constantly remains challenged and working hard for you.

7. *Exercise.* Discover your body type, and then follow the guidelines given in the revised and expanded version of *Bloodtypes, Bodytypes, and You.*

8. *Find a buddy.* Support is always helpful. You can coach each other through the program. You don't have to be the same blood type.

9. *Drink plenty of water.* Oftentimes we mistake our bodies' need for more water for hunger pains. Try drinking a small glass of water when you think you're hungry.

10. *Chew . . . chew . . . chew.* Eat slowly, and chew your food very well. This will aid the digestion process.

11. *Put your fork down.* Put your fork down between bites. This will slow down your meal consumption time and enable you to actually allow your body to feel full.

12. *Remember that this program is a "lifestyle change."* It is not a diet. Diets are temporary. Lifestyle changes are a lifelong practice.

13. *Take it easy.* Be patient with yourself. Any new regimen will take some getting used to.

14. *Take time for yourself.* Do something you enjoy at least ONCE a week. Doing something good for yourself helps you to remember that you are alive and worth the investment of having better health, a fuller life, and a deeper commitment to yourself.

## Tips for Dining Out

1. *Have a game plan.* First and foremost know what the structure of your meal will look like *before* you go into a restaurant. We all have a tendency to glaze over when we see the glossy menus the waiter hands to us. For example, the components of your dinner should look like this:

   - Lean protein the size of your palm (blood-type appropriate)
   - 1 serving dark leafy green vegetables

- 1 serving other vegetable

- 1 serving carbohydrate (optional)

I usually will go to a restaurant that serves fish or steak. A meal out for me might consist of a tuna or beef steak, sautéed spinach, a side salad or a side order of O-appropriate vegetables, and wild rice.

2. *Ask questions; special requests are OK.* Ask your server what is in the dish you are considering if you are unsure. Most servers are happy to provide such information. If you would like a change to the dish, within reason, do not hesitate to ask. Most establishments are used to accommodating their customers' special dietary needs.

3. *Remove bread from the table.* There is no need to tempt yourself.

4. *Place a glass of water in front of you.* Drink after you eat, not while you eat. It may seem difficult, but if you chew thoroughly, it will be a snap.

5. *Choose desserts carefully.* If your dessert craving kicks in, try my 80/20 rule, but in most cases after eating a full meal, who is still hungry? Forgo the dessert in the restaurant, and have something you have prepared yourself when you get home.

6. *Enjoy your dinner companions.* Focus on the people you are with rather than the food. After all, part of a good meal out is the company.

## In Conclusion

My desire for writing this book has been to communicate, in a reader-friendly way, valuable information that pertains specifically to you as a person with blood type A. This book can serve as the next best thing to having your own personal nutrition and fitness coach. I have given you the best I can on paper to get you started in the right direction and ultimately to help you reach your goals—the rest is up to you!

I hope something in this book has motivated you and perhaps even challenged your former way of thinking about yourself, your health, and others. Discovering the connection between your genetics and how your body functions should overwhelm you with the realization that you have been wonderfully and incredibly made. You are not just another body on this planet. You possess a uniqueness that sets you apart from anyone else; you are worthy of the best.

Your journey to a healthier lifestyle will not begin by accident but through deliberate actions. Your body has not been designed to be idle; it is designed to be physically active. So, you must determine that there is no such thing as living a sedentary lifestyle any longer. Your mind can be clear and alert so it can function at its maximum capacity when you eat correctly and exercise regularly. When it is free of negative thoughts like anger, jealousy, hatred, anxiety, doubt, fear, lust, and self-centeredness, your body will begin the healing process and prolong the onset of diseases. In the world around you, you will find people who are attracted to you by the example you live, not by what you say.

Though our paths may never cross, may our commitment to a healthier, more energetic life be the common ground we walk. Continue on the journey, stay the course, stay positive, and remember—you are an inspiration in transition!

Focus on the purpose, not the task!

# Appendix A

# NUTRITION SUPPORT IDEAS

## Colon Health

### Inner Out: Fourteen-day colon cleansing and detoxifying system

The Inner Out Colon Cleansing and Detoxifying System is designed to generate a progressive cleansing effect on your body for fourteen days. It does this in three phases: Phase 1, preparation—kills parasites and breaks up mucous buildup. Phase 2, cleansing—scrubs and cleans the colon. Phase 3, restoration—restores normal colon function with added probiotics.

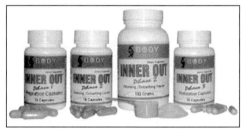

## Enzymes

### Digestive Enzymes

This digestive enzyme matrix is loaded with a complete line of enzymes to meet any shortage of enzyme production that may be missing in your digestive system. Each capsule contains a matrix of enzymes that provide the specificity of enzymatic action for every food group, creating a greater capacity for better digestion, assimilation, and uptake of nutrition from the foods you eat.

## Vitamins

### A.M./P.M. Multivitamins

This is a daily multivitamin supplement for blood types A, B, AB, and O. Each formula contains vitamins, minerals, antioxidants, and herbs specifically formulated to meet the nutritional requirements of each blood type.

## Trace Minerals

### ConcenTrace

These are liquid trace minerals. Our bodies do not manufacture them! One of the secrets to good health and longevity is found in the soil—trace minerals! This source of organic trace minerals has a similar complement of precious organic trace minerals. We are made from dust of the earth, and this dust, our own soils, is greatly depleted. ConcenTrace liquid trace mineral supplementation is a very necessary and healthy choice.

## Calcium

### Coral Calcium

Calcium is a priceless organic mineral and essential for the function of every organ and gland. It is also imperative for balancing the blood and tissue pH in the body. Calcium is the major mineral our body needs in abundance, yet it is the most difficult mineral to absorb. Coral calcium, marine grade, imported from Okinawa, Japan, with magnesium and vitamin $D_3$ (cholecalciferol) is formulated to promote proper assimilation in the body.

## PROTEIN

### Body Genetics Protein Shakes and Thin Tastic Protein Bars

Protein is essential for your body. Your body could not function without it. You need enough protein on a daily basis. Other than food sources, you should supplement your diet with a shake or bar as an afternoon pick-me-up or midmorning grab-and-go. Whatever your preference, be certain to include enough protein throughout every day.

## WATER

### Alkaline water

You can go without eating for days, even weeks, but you cannot go very long without water. Every cell in your body is craving the quenching effect of hydration. Revitalize your cellular strength, bring more life into your skin, and supply your body with organic minerals that protect it from disease and chemical imbalance with every ounce of water you drink—drink alkaline water.

## ANTIAGING

### Homeopathic HGH, orally absorbed

To roll back the clock is impossible, but to slow down or reverse the negative effects associated with the aging process is possible. By supplementing with HGH, replacing what time and nature can no longer produce, you can enjoy sleeping better, more energy, smoother-looking skin, lower cholesterol, lower percent of body fat, and feelings of youthfulness. You once had enough HGH; now be certain that you still do through supplementation.

There are many other nutritional supplements I could have listed, but for our purpose of covering the major nutritional needs, I feel these will go a long way to filling your health pack.

## ORGANIC PRODUCTS ONLINE

www.organicfruitsandnuts.com
www.edenfoods.com
www.kalustyans.com

You can also e-mail the following for information:

rosebock@flex.net
magedson@unicomp.net
slanker@neto.com
jmoseley@webwide.net

## CHEMICAL-FREE MEAT AND GRAINS

### Organic meats

Coleman Natural Products, Inc., 1767 Denver West Blvd., Suite 200m Golden, CO 80401, (800) 442-8666

### Specialty meat and poultry

D'Artagnan, 280 Wilson Ave., Newark, NJ 07105, (800) 327-8246

## Spelt flour and pastas

Purity Foods, 2871 W. Jolly Rd., Okemos, MI 48864, (517) 351-9231.

## CHILDREN'S HEALTH

### Dump the Junk

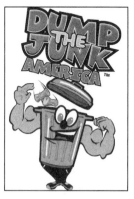

For kids under construction, Dr. Christiano has developed the Dump the Junk curriculum for grades K–12 that includes nutrition, exercise, and attitude. He applies his "whole child" approach for helping our kids be physically and mentally fit and more academically sound. For more information, please go to www.dumpthejunkamerica.com.

For all Body Genetics products, go to:
www.bodyredesigning.com
Or call
(800) 259-2639

## Appendix B

# MEAL-PLANNER CHART

| DAY | Breakfast | Lunch | Dinner | |
|-----|-----------|-------|--------|---|
| **1** | Snack | Snack | Snack | |
| **2** | Snack | Snack | Snack | |
| **3** | Snack | Snack | Snack | |
| **4** | Snack | Snack | Snack | |
| **5** | Snack | Snack | Snack | |
| **6** | Snack | Snack | Snack | |
| **7** | Snack | Snack | Snack | |

NOTE: Add your chosen option number to the small boxes for ready reference. Write the name of each option in the space provided.

# Appendix C

# THERMOBLAST WEIGHT-LOSS MEAL REPLACEMENTS

## Body Genetics Meal Replacement Bar

*Body Genetics Meal Replacement Bar* creates a thermoblast when it comes to losing weight. It is formulated to increase the body's ability to burn calories. It comes in delicious dark chocolate and serves as the perfect meal replacement for weight-loss enhancement. It is loaded with over seventy antioxidants for cellular and cardiovascular protection.

Benefits: It stimulates the metabolism and enhances weight loss, causing the body to use fat for energy. It is filling, delicious, it cuts sugar cravings, and it is satisfying. It keeps you from skipping meals, which is detrimental to basal metabolic rate (BMR).

## Body Genetics Strawberry-Filled Cookies (also Blueberry-Filled Cookies)

*Body Genetics Strawberry-Filled Cookies* have been formulated to serve as a meal replacement or snack. The awesomely delicious taste makes weight loss fun, tasty, and satisfying. Each cookie is naturally prepared and has a unique proprietary blend of natural ingredients that work synergistically to stimulate the metabolism for weight loss.

Benefits: The cookies aid the metabolism for additional calorie burning and satisfy cravings for sweets. They are a good fat-burning meal replacement or snack.

### Body Genetics Energy Booster/Fat Burner tablets

*Body Genetics Energy Booster/Fat Burner* tablets are a nonephedrine thermogenic supplement designed to enhance weight loss. Each tablet has a unique proprietary blend of natural ingredients that work synergistically to stimulate the metabolism for weight loss and increased energy. Tablets cause no adverse side effects commonly associated with weight loss and energy products that use ma huang and/or ephedra.

Benefits: The tablets burn calories, suppress appetite, improve performance, and increase energy and mental alertness.

For further information on ordering these and other Body Genetics nutritional products, contact us at:

Body Redesigning by Joseph Christiano
www.bodyredesigning.com
(800) 259-2639

# Appendix D

## THERMOBLAST TWELVE-WEEK WEIGHT LOSS PROGRAM

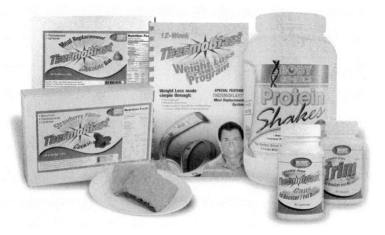

### Jump-Start Components

- Thirty-two-page booklet that includes the weight-loss concept; instructions; and seven varieties of breakfast, lunch, dinner, and snacks that are compatible for ALL blood types

- Thirty-day progressive walking program for gradual fitness conditioning

- One box (14) Thermoblast Strawberry Cookies

- One box (14) Thermoblast Chocolate Meal Replacement Bars

- Thermoblast Energy/Metabolism Booster (60 caps) or TRIM (caffeine free)

- French Vanilla or Dutch Chocolate Protein Shake (30 servings)

Home Blood Typing Kits are also available. All weight-loss products are available individually.

For further information on ordering these and other Body Genetics Nutritional products, contact us at:

Body Redesigning by Joseph Christiano
www.bodyredesigning.com
(800) 259-2639

# Appendix E

# HEALTH AND FITNESS COACHING AND SERVICES

### Fork in the Road—the Road Map to Redesigning a New You

Fork in the Road is a dynamic motivational Health and Fitness Life Coaching DVD series designed to assist the individual who is ready to make healthy lifestyle changes. Professional health and fitness trainer and life coach Dr. Joseph Christiano implements three fundamental components —attitude, diet, and exercise— 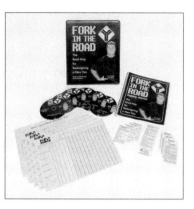 for successfully reaching your fullest potential.

As your life coach and personal trainer, Dr. Joe teaches you how to overcome negative influences, make positive decisions, and rediscover your personal worth by challenging your mental attitude. While developing the correct mental attitude you will learn how to reach your physical genetic potential for weight loss, disease-free living, and maximum health. Dr. Joe teaches how to individualize and be most accurate with food and exercise by factoring in your unique genetic individuality.

Included in the series are the following DVDs:

- DVD 1 - Introduction to Series
- DVD 2 - Redesigning Your Attitude

- DVD 3 - Redesigning Your Diet

- DVD 4 - Redesigning Your Exercise

- DVD 5 - Redesigning Your Shape (Women)

- DVD 6 - Redesigning Your Workout (Men)

- Mapping Journal

- Food Cards

- Live online monthly coaching for teaching, motivation, and accountability with Dr. Christiano (optional)

For further information on ordering these and other Body Genetics products, contact us at:

Body Redesigning by Joseph Christiano
www.bodyredesigning.com
800-259-2639

# Appendix F

# SERVICES AND BENEFITS

## PIP—Personalized Illness Profile "Eliminate Illness by Eradicating the Root Cause!"

### Problem: ILLNESS

If you are like most people, you may very well be dealing with some sort of health issue that is disrupting your state of well-being and robbing you of the quality of life you are seeking. And you are probably very frustrated by the lack of results. This is true because you have been shown how to treat the symptoms, not the root causes.

Addressing illnesses has become a vicious cycle of identifying symptoms, symptom stomping with medications, and continued poor health…until now!

### Solution: ERADICATION

Once an illness, disorder, or sickness has been determined, the next step is to identify and eradicate the root cause of the condition. Seek and destroy the root cause of your illnesses, and you will restore your health.

PIP is an extensive health evaluation, which includes all ten body systems. The evaluation will expose which system(s) in your body is compromised and by what root cause. Some of these root causes can be anything from a parasite such as mold, fungus, slime mold, or worms, or environmental toxins such as chlorine, dyes, or other solvents. Other root causes may be food allergies and/or hormonal imbalances.

## HEALTHY PARTNER

Being a health-conscious person makes becoming a Healthy Partner a natural fit at www.bodyredesigning.com. As a Healthy Partner you receive 30 percent off of all purchases, as well as additional benefits such as our e-newsletter, savings on shipping and handling costs, plus free access to our online Health and Fitness Coaching sessions with Dr. Christiano. Visit our Web site at www.bodyredesigning.com for more information about PIP and/or becoming a Healthy Partner.

# Notes

## INTRODUCTION

1. Weight-Control Information Network (WIN), "Statistics Related to Overweight and Obesity," National Institute of Diabetes and Digestive and Kidney Diseases (NIDDK), http://win.niddk.nih.gov/statistics/index.htm (accessed December 18, 2007).

2. Rob Wilkins and Mike O'Hearn, "Obesity! Public Enemy Number One," *Natural Muscle*, January 2000, 28.

## CHAPTER 1

## BLOOD TYPES: YOUR FOUNDATION FOR HEALTH

1. Jesper L. Anderson, Peter Schjerling, and Bengt Saltin, "Muscle, Genes and Athletic Performance," *Scientific American*, September 2000, 49–55.

2. Ibid.

3. "Diabetes Risk Written on a Gene," *USA Today*, August 28, 2000, 6D.

4. Associated Press, "Discovery Opens Door to Treat Obesity, Diabetes," *Orlando Sentinel*, September 20, 2000, A3.

5. Nancy McVicar, "Genome Work Spurs Grant for Miami School," *Orlando Sentinel*, August 30, 2000, D5.

6. Jonathan Safarti, "Blood Types and Their Origins (Answering the Critics)," *TJ: Journal of Creation* 11, no. 1 (April 1997): 31–32, http://creation.com/images/pdfs/tj/j11_1/j11_1_31-32.pdf (accessed May 3, 2010).

7. Michael Denton, *Evolution: A Theory in Crisis* (Bethesda, MD: Adler and Adler, 1985), 16, as quoted in a dissertation by Dr. Carl E. Baugh, "Conventional Explanation for Human Antiquities in Question," http://www.creationevidence.org/carlbaugh/diss1.htm (accessed January 15, 2008).

## CHAPTER 2
### BLOOD TYPE AND NUTRITION

1. Steven M. Weissberg and Joseph Christiano, *The Answer Is in Your Bloodtype* (Lake Mary, FL: Personal Nutrition USA, 1999), 57.

## CHAPTER 4
### TYPE A: EVERYTHING YOU NEED TO KNOW

1. Wessberg and Christiano, *The Answer Is in Your Bloodtype*, 37–43.

2. Ibid., 154.

3. Ann Louise Gittleman with James Templeton and Candace Versace, *Your Body Knows Best* (New York: Pocket Books, a div. of Simon and Schuster, Inc., 1996), 126–127.

## CHAPTER 7
### INDIVIDUALIZED EATING PLAN FOR TYPE A

1. Beneficial, neutral, and avoid foods lists have been adapted and expanded from the following sources: Peter J. D'Adamo, *Eat Right for Your Blood Type* (New York: Putnam Publ. Group, 1997); Steven M. Weissberg and Joseph Christiano, *The Answer Is in Your Bloodtype* (Lake Mary, FL: Personal Nutrition USA, 1999).

## CHAPTER 8
### PICK-A-MEAL RECIPES FOR TYPE A

1. Molly O'Neill, *New York Cookbook* (n.p., n.d.), 326–327.

2. The Moosewood Collective, *Moosewood Restaurant Low-Fat Favorites* (n.p., 1996), 289.

3. Adapted with slight changes from *Prevention's The Healthy Cook* by the editors of *Prevention Magazine* Health Books (Emmaus, PA: Rodale Press, Inc., 1997), 255.

4. Adapted with slight changes from *The Kripalu Cookbook* by Atma Joanne Levitt (Lee, MA: Berkshire House Publishers, 1995), 30.

5. Adapted with slight changes from *Vegetarian Times Complete Cookbook* by Vegetarian Times, Inc. (New York: Macmillan, 1995), 403.

6. Adapted with slight changes from *The Self-Healing Cookbook,* 7th edition, by Kristina Turner (Vashon Island, WA: Earthtones Press, 1998), 113.

## CHAPTER 9
### NUTRITIONAL SUPPLEMENTS FOR TYPE A

1. "Negative Thoughts Make You Ill," *Medical News Today,* http://www.medicalnewstoday.com/articles/4227.php (accessed May 5, 2010).